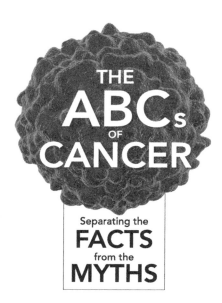

THE
ABCs
OF
CANCER

Separating the
FACTS
from the
MYTHS

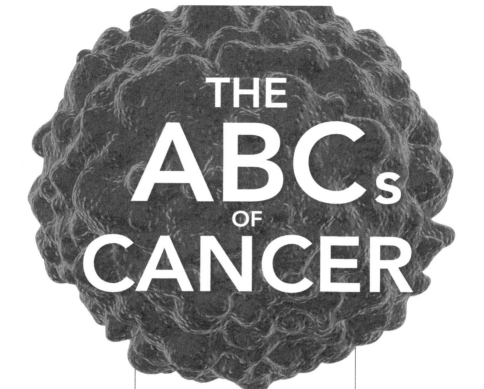

THE
ABCs
OF
CANCER

Separating the
FACTS
from the
MYTHS

Meshach Asare-Werehene

The University of Ottawa, Canada
Ottawa Hospital Research Institute, Canada

World Scientific

NEW JERSEY · LONDON · SINGAPORE · BEIJING · SHANGHAI · HONG KONG · TAIPEI · CHENNAI · TOKYO

Published by

World Scientific Publishing Co. Pte. Ltd.
5 Toh Tuck Link, Singapore 596224
USA office: 27 Warren Street, Suite 401-402, Hackensack, NJ 07601
UK office: 57 Shelton Street, Covent Garden, London WC2H 9HE

Library of Congress Control Number: 2020938740

British Library Cataloguing-in-Publication Data
A catalogue record for this book is available from the British Library.

THE ABCs OF CANCER
Separating the Facts from the Myths

ISBN 978-981-121-225-3 (hardcover)
ISBN 978-981-121-226-0 (ebook for institutions)
ISBN 978-981-121-227-7 (ebook for individuals)

For any available supplementary material, please visit
https://www.worldscientific.com/worldscibooks/10.1142/11606#t=suppl

Typeset by Stallion Press
Email: enquiries@stallionpress.com

Printed in Singapore

Preface

Cancer continues to plague the lives of many. Although much effort has been channeled into its diagnosis and management as well as discovery of new treatment modalities, the battle seems far from being won. The name cancer is not only scary but also very complex. The complexity of cancer makes it not appealing to the nonscientific audience to read and comprehend any article about cancer research. There are many news articles about cancer research; however, some of these articles either are difficult to understand by nonscientific audience or contain fallacious statements. There have been many published cancer myths being purported as facts, creating fear and panic among the populace. In this book, the author carefully separates cancer myths from the facts through the use of scientific evidence. The chapters are easy to read and comprehend irrespective of your educational background. This book also addresses societal lifestyles that have long been linked to cancer risks. This book is a must-have resource not only for science-inclined people but also for anyone with an interest in knowing about cancer.

Contents

Chapter 1

Introduction to Cancer

Cancer continues to be one of the deadliest diseases regardless of the efforts channeled into research. Although some cancers such as melanoma (cancer of the skin) have seen some improvement in patients' survival, others such as ovarian, prostate, and brain cancers still lag in terms of effective treatment and overall patients' survival. There have been new treatment alternatives; however, little clinical significance has been seen. There are currently studies in the areas of early detection, precision medicine, and effective management with the hope that cancer will be tackled efficiently.

Although cancer developments mostly result from altered genes, lifestyles and the environment could also have a major influence. Eating a well-balanced diet, regular exercises, avoiding smoking and alcohol, and decreased exposure to carcinogenic substances and radiations may decrease one's risk of developing cancer. Although one might have inherited an altered gene, living a healthy lifestyle will lessen the individual's chances of developing the cancer associated with the altered gene (Fig. 1).

Cancer is believed to be a collection of diseases that manifest in the body and start from the cells. When the genes regulating the activities of the cells are altered, the cells grow uncontrollably and overshadow the immune system. Once the immune system is shut

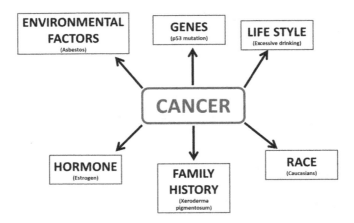

Fig. 1.   Contributing factors for cancer development

down, they have the opportunity to move from their original starting place into other organs, which is termed metastasis. This usually occurs when the cancer cells secrete substances that are able to induce the formation of new blood vessels to make their movement easier, a condition referred to as angiogenesis. Thus developing treatments against metastasis and angiogenesis could help in controlling the growth of cancer cells and be helpful to patients.

There are different types of cancers and they are mostly determined by their origin such as carcinoma (cancer that originates from epithelial cells), sarcoma (bone and soft tissues), leukemia (blood-forming cells), melanoma (melanocytes — cells that give the skin its color), lymphoma (lymphocytes — disease-fighting cells such as T cells and B cells), multiple myeloma (plasma cells — another type of immune cells), germ cell tumors (cells that form sperms and eggs), and neuroendocrine tumors (cells that produce hormones). Each of these cancer types also has different subtypes of cancers that could be further subdivided. This gives some picture of how complex cancer is and why finding treatments becomes extremely difficult. It is also worth knowing that no two cancers are the same. For example, two breast cancer patients might not respond to the same treatment regimen due to lots of reasons such as different stage of the cancers, different gene mutations or drivers, lifestyle, immune system makeup, and other related medical complications. Thus, there is the move to patronizing precision medicine where the treatments are well tailored to each patient based on their tumor profile and clinical history.

The immune system is a key player in cancer treatment and over the decade, massive studies have unveiled the possibilities of harnessing the immune system to fight cancer. This is known as cancer immunotherapy or immuno-oncology. Scientists in the field believe when the immune systems are fully functional, they automatically fight the tumor cells; however, when they are dysfunctional, it's unable to eliminate the tumor cells. Thus, the tumor cells outgrow the immune cells and disarm them. Knowing this concept, they believe, reengineering the affected immune cells to their functional state will provide some therapeutic effects. This has led to the development of checkpoint blockers (antibodies) that release the brakes on T cells (a type of immune cell) to attack cancer cells. These antibodies have been approved by FDA and are being used in clinics to treat melanoma and other solid tumors. It is believed using this approach will prevent chemotherapy-induced toxicities and produce an effective alternative to fighting cancer.

There have been new studies that have resulted in discovering approaches used in the early detection of cancer, revealing target markers for effective treatments as well as management of patients. Most of these approaches are made possible by the technological advancements in the field of artificial intelligence, machine learning, gene editing, and nanotechnology. With these, there is some level of assurance that the fight against cancer will be a victorious one.

Due to the complex nature of cancer, there have been lots of myths dumped on the Internet, which usually bring fear and panic to the masses. Most people buy into these hoax contents and are not able to live a happy life. Although cancer is complex, knowing the facts supported with scientific evidence could lessen the fear and help improve the lives of people. Finding the right resources to sieve the facts from the myths is very challenging. Most companies or media outlets often support biased reports that will help sustain their businesses and hence the consumers are the ones that suffer at the end of the day. For example, a sugar business is likely to support a report that will favor the business and direct the blame to an oil or fat industry. With such biases going on, consumers are torn apart and do not know the facts from the myths.

Here, well-proven scientific evidences are used to sieve the facts from the myths in simple terms that are easily understandable by readers regardless of their scientific background. Complex mechanisms and scientific studies are broken down in lay terms without losing their relevance.

Bibliography

Altmann DM. (2018). A Nobel Prize-worthy pursuit: Cancer immunology and harnessing immunity to tumour neoantigens. *Immunology, 155*(3), 283–284. doi:10.1111/imm.13008.

Baan R, Straif K, Grosse Y, *et al.* (2007). Carcinogenicity of alcoholic beverages. *The Lancet Oncology, 8*(4), 292–293.

Bingham SA, Day NE, Luben R, *et al.* (2003). Dietary fibre in food and protection against colorectal cancer in the European Prospective Investigation into Cancer and Nutrition (EPIC): An observational study. *Lancet, 361*(9368), 1496–1501.

Bouvard V, Loomis D, Guyton KZ, *et al.* (2015). Carcinogenicity of consumption of red and processed meat. *The Lancet Oncology, 16*(16), 1599–1600.

de la Cruz-Merino L, Chiesa M, Caballero R, *et al.* (2017). Breast cancer immunology and immunotherapy: Current status and future perspectives. *International Review of Cell and Molecular Biology, 331*, 1–53. doi:10.1016/bs.ircmb.2016.09.008.

Doll R, Peto R. (1981). The causes of cancer: Quantitative estimates of avoidable risks of cancer in the United States today. *Journal of the National Cancer Institute, 66*(6), 1191–1308.

Goetze TO. (2015). Gallbladder carcinoma: Prognostic factors and therapeutic options. *World Journal of Gastroenterology, 21*(43), 12211–12217. doi:10.3748/wjg.v21.i43.12211.

Huncharek M, Kupelnick B. (2005). Personal use of hair dyes and the risk of bladder cancer: Results of a meta-analysis. *Public Health Reports (Washington, D.C.: 1974), 120*(1), 31–38.

Ijsselsteijn ME, Sanz-Pamplona R, Hermitte F, de Miranda NFCC. (2019). Colorectal cancer: A paradigmatic model for cancer immunology and immunotherapy. *Molecular Aspects of Medicine, 69*, 123–129. doi:10.1016/j. mam.2019.05.003.

Latikka P, Pukkala E, Vihko V. (1998). Relationship between the risk of breast cancer and physical activity. An epidemiological perspective. *Sports Medicine, 26*(3), 133–143.

Lyytinen HK, Dyba T, Ylikorkala O, Pukkala EI. (2010). A case-control study on hormone therapy as a risk factor for breast cancer in Finland: Intrauterine system carries a risk as well. *International Journal of Cancer, 126*(2), 483–489.

Parkin DM, Boyd L, Walker LC. (2011). The fraction of cancer attributable to lifestyle and environmental factors in the UK in 2010. *British Journal of Cancer, 105*, S77–81.

Thorsson V, Gibbs DL, Brown SD, *et al.* (2018). The immune landscape of cancer. *Immunity, 48*(4), 812–830.e14. doi:10.1016/j.immuni.2018.03.023

Turati F, Pelucchi C, Galeone C, Decarli A, La Vecchia C. (2014). Personal hair dye use and bladder cancer: A meta-analysis. *Annals of Epidemiology, 24*(2), 151–159.

Xue F, Willett WC, Rosner BA, Hankinson SE, Michels KB. (2011). Cigarette smoking and the incidence of breast cancer. *Archives of Internal Medicine, 171*(2), 125–133.

Chapter 2

Your Genes Are Big Players in Cancer Development

Genes act like molecular switches that control the behavior of cells such as dividing, growing, and dying. They carry special instructions that enable the cells to produce proteins for their daily work. When these genes are normal, they help the body evade diseases such as cancer. However, when there are changes in the genes, they predispose the body to the development of cancer and other chronic diseases. These changes are called mutations and could cause malfunctioning of proteins, which ultimately affect the normal behavior of the cells in the body. Gene mutations result in the elimination or amplification of protein functions, leading to the uncontrolled growth of normal cells and tumor development. Some of the types of cancer-related mutations are missense (where there is a change in the amino acids sequence of the protein), nonsense (where the protein produced is shorter than usual), frameshift (where the mutation produces a protein that is different in size and function compared with the normal protein), and chromosomal rearrangements (where a piece of the chromosome is broken, deleted, or moved to other parts of the chromosome; the pieces could also be flipped to assume a different position).

Genetic alterations could be inherited from parents and transferred to the next generation. Usually, these are termed as germ line mutations since the altered genes are located in the reproductive cells of the sperms and eggs, also called germ cells. Inherited genetic mutations account for about 5–10% of all cancers and can predispose an individual as a high risk for future cancer development. Individuals with such mutations stand a higher chance of developing cancer; however, it does not necessarily mean they will have cancer. Familial cancers are distinct from inherited cancers. Familial cancers have higher occurrence in families more than would be expected by chance. These cancers are mostly related to the lifestyle of families such as place of stay, food, physical activity, chemical usage, and working environment.

Beside inherited genetic alterations, there are other mutations that are acquired or influenced by the environment. They are known as acquired, somatic, or sporadic genetic alterations. This usually occurs due to old age or when an individual comes into contact with carcinogenic compounds, radiations, tobacco smoking, and ultraviolet rays from the sun. These mutations do not happen at once but over time in an individual's life (Fig. 1).

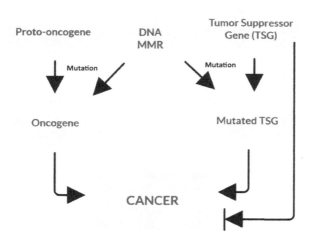

Fig. 1. Genetic alterations can result in cancer

There are three groups of genes that are implicated in cancer development.

1. *Oncogenes*: These are sets of mutated genes that drive cells to divide uncontrollably resulting in the development of cancer. These genes behave like switches that are always turned on. There are subclasses of normal genes called proto-oncogenes that are usually turned off. Once these proto-oncogenes are mutated, they behave like oncogenes and drive cells to divide uncontrollably. Examples of oncogenes are *PKB* (protein kinase B; has been implicated in ovarian, breast, colon, head-and-neck, and colon cancers), *HER2* (human epidermal growth factor receptor 2; has been implicated in breast, stomach, and esophageal cancers), *KRAS* (originally identified from Kirsten RAt Sarcoma virus and has been shown to be involved in lung, pancreas, and colorectal cancers), *BRAF* (mutations of this gene have been indicated in liver, kidney, colorectal, melanoma, brain, and lung cancers), *EGFR* (human epidermal growth factor receptor; mostly mutated in patients with non-small cell lung cancer), and *GSN* (gelsolin; recent studies have shown that GSN is highly implicated in ovarian, prostate, head-and-neck, and lung cancers).

2. *Tumor suppressor genes* (*TSGs*): These are normal genes that prevent cells from dividing rapidly to avoid cancer development as well as help repair errors during DNA damage. Also, they are able to tell cells when to die, a process known as programmed cell death (apoptosis). Most of the times, these genes are turned on to put rapidly dividing cells under control. Once mutated, they are turned off and thus unable to put brakes on rapidly dividing cells. Under such unfortunate conditions, cells divide rapidly and uncontrollably, resulting in cancer. Some of the well-studied TSGs are *RB1* gene (retinoblastoma gene; the first TSG to be identified and mostly mutated in human retinoblastoma — an eye cancer that originates from the retina), BRCA genes (*BRCA1* and *2*; mostly mutated in breast and ovarian cancers; mutation of these genes serves as a high-risk factor for pancreatic, prostate, and

male breast cancers), *TP53* gene (this gene is mutated in about 50% of all cancers and thus making it the most common TSG), *PTEN* (mutations have been identified in thyroid, breast, ovarian, and endometrial cancers), and *APC* (adenomatous polyposis coli gene; *APC* mutations increase a person's risk of developing colon and pancreatic cancers).

3. *DNA mismatch repair genes (MMR)*: During active cell division, errors are generated in the DNA and are repaired by the MMRs. Mutations in MMRs prevent correction of these errors in TSGs and oncogenes and thus resulting in cancer. MMR mutations predispose individuals to ovarian, endometrial, stomach, colorectal, and bladder cancers. Examples of such genes are *MSH2*, *MSH6*, *MLH1*, and *PMS2*.

There are several clues to indicate if a cancer is a result of an inherited mutated gene or not. One or more cases of childhood cancers, a rare type of cancer in the family, developing cancer in both organs (such as breast, kidneys, and eyes), multiple cancers (breast and ovarian cancers), and same cancers among family members could suggest a mutated gene has been inherited.

Although one might not be able to control the inheritance of a mutated gene, there are some measures to take that will help decrease your risk of developing cancers. Knowing your family history, genetic screening, avoiding smoking and carcinogenic agents, regular medical checkups, healthy diets, adapting an active lifestyle, and preventive surgery of a high-risk organ (such as breast or ovary) could potentially lower risks of developing cancers.

Family cancer syndromes are rare conditions caused by inheriting a mutated gene. Although these syndromes are not cancers themselves, they increase the risks of developing cancer. Knowing your family history as well as genetic screening could be beneficial. These syndromes are mostly associated with families where childhood cancers are frequently diagnosed and multiple cancers are found in one individual (breast and ovarian). Examples of family cancer syndromes are xeroderma pigmentosum (XP), Wiskott–Aldrich syndrome, Ataxia-telangiectasia, Bloom syndrome, basal cell nevus syndrome, Beckwith–Wiedemann syndrome, Carney complex, Gardner syndrome, familial atypical multiple mole melanoma (FAMMM) syndrome, familial adenomatous polyposis (FAP), Cowden syndrome, Li–Fraumeni syndrome, Lynch syndrome, hereditary retinoblastoma, hereditary breast and ovarian cancer (HBOC) syndrome, Von Hippel–Lindau (VHL) syndrome, Turcot syndrome, multiple endocrine neoplasia (MEN), Peutz–Jeghers syndrome, neurofibromatosis type 1, and Werner syndrome.

Genetic screening is a clinical test that looks out for alterations in chromosomes, genes, or proteins that are linked to cancer or syndromes that increase your risk of developing cancer. Genetic testing is not only used in the field of cancer, but also in other diseases related to genetic changes. Before this test, your family doctor together with a genetic counselor will let the individual understand how the test works, the samples needed, how altered genes result in cancer, benefits and drawbacks of the test, and how the results might impact the family. Informed consent will then be received from the individual before the test is finally carried out by a licensed and qualified medical professional. The samples mostly used for genetic testing are blood, saliva, urine, tissue, or skin. Any of these samples carry enough DNA that could be used for the analysis. Genetic testing is conducted using different approaches including biochemical tests (where enzymes and proteins are analyzed), molecular testing (which investigates mutations in genes and chromosomes), and whole genome testing (analyses the entire genetic makeup of an individual). Recently, there is another means of doing this test where companies sell genetic testing kits directly to the client and the clients return the kits with the sample for analysis via courier. This method is known as direct-to-consumer (DTC) testing. With this approach, the client does not go through any genetic counseling or a professional healthcare giver. Clients must therefore be extremely careful when dealing with such companies. Although genetic testing is very helpful, it's however not conclusive. Testing positive for a genetic mutation does not automatically mean you will develop cancer. Likewise, a negative result does not mean you won't develop cancer. This result together with your medical history will provide your healthcare givers the best information to enable them to provide you with effective preventive care or therapeutic options.

Genes could also be modified by a process called epigenetics rather than mutation of the genetic code itself. Such modifications could either switch the gene on or off, a condition that affects the behavior of cells.

1. *DNA methylation*: This epigenetic change involves the addition of a methyl group to the DNA. This inactivates the function of the gene and makes it unable to code for the protein it's originally intended for.
2. *Histone modification*: DNA is wrapped around histones in order to form a chromosome. The addition or deletion of an acetyl group can either activate or deactivate that part of the chromosome. These modifications can also affect the behavior of cells irrespective of genetic mutations.
3. *RNA interference*: Recent studies have shown that some small forms of RNAs can interrupt genetic expressions as well as the normal functioning of histones and DNA.

Beside the above stated and well-studied genes, alterations of other genes have been implicated in a plethora of cancers such as epithelial ovarian cancer (*GSN, ABC transporters, PRC1, LRRC46, CHMP4C, HAUS6,* and *KANSL1*), prostate cancer (*BAZ2A, SMAD4, CDKN2A, ARID1A, KDM6A, PREX2,* and *ROBO2*), and breast cancer (*IGFBP5* and *ZNF365*).

More often than not, there are many instances where a couple of genes are involved in the development of a particular cancer such as ovarian cancer. In such circumstances, a multifactorial approach to treatment provides better and efficient results compared with monotherapies (single treatments) due to the heterogeneous nature of the tumor. Thus, targeting just one gene will provide less therapeutic success to patients. Also, multipanel genetic screening will aid in the detection of an array of altered genes responsible for a particular cancer.

Our genes play a key role in the development of diseases especially cancer. However, other environmental factors such as lifestyle, diet, exposure to carcinogens, and other factors could impact the behavior of genes. Knowing your family history, taking a genetic screening, and engaging a genetic counselor could be beneficial in deciding your risk status for cancer.

Bibliography

Ahearn TU, Peisch S, Pettersson A, *et al.* (2018). Expression of IGF/insulin receptor in prostate cancer tissue and progression to lethal disease. *Carcinogenesis, 39*(12), 1431–1437. doi:10.1093/carcin/bgy112.

American Cancer Society. (2014, June 23). *Family Cancer Syndromes.* Retrieved from http://www.cancer.org/cancer/cancercauses/genetic-sandcancer/heredity-and-cancer.

American Cancer Society. (2014, June 25). *Genes and Cancer.* Retrieved from http://www.cancer.org/acs/groups/cid/documents/webcontent/002550-pdf.pdf.

American Society of Clinical Oncology. (2016). *Hereditary Cancer-related Syndromes.* Retrieved from http://www.cancer.net/navigating-cancer-care/cancer-basics/genetics/hereditary-cancer-related-syndromes.

Bahcall O. (2013). Common variation and heritability estimates for breast, ovarian and prostate cancers. *Nature Genetics.* Retrieved from http://www.nature.com/icogs/primer/common-variation-and-heritability-esti-mates-for-breast-ovarian-and-prostate-cancers/.

Bailey J, Hendley A, Lafaro K, *et al.* (2016). p53 mutations cooperate with oncogenic Kras to promote adenocarcinoma from pancreatic ductal cells. *Oncogene, 35*, 4282–4288. doi:10.1038/onc.2015.441.

Darabi H, McCue K, Beesley J, *et al.* (2015). Polymorphisms in a putative enhancer at the 10q21.2 breast cancer risk locus regulate NRBF2 expression. *American Journal of Human Genetics, 97*(1), 22–34. doi:10.1016/j.ajhg.2015.05.002.

Davidson NE, Armstrong SA, Coussens LM, *et al.* (2016). AACR cancer progress report 2016. *Clinical Cancer Research, 22*(Suppl. 19), S1–S137. Retrieved from http://cancerprogressreport.org/2016/Documents/CPR2016.pdf.

Findlay GM, Daza RM, Martin B, *et al.* (2018). Accurate classification of BRCA1 variants with saturation genome editing. *Nature, 562*(7726), 217–222.

Garassino M. (2013). *Personalised Cancer Medicine: An ESMO Guide for Patients.* Retrieved from https://www.esmo.org/content/download/20122/337223/file/ESMO-Patient-Guide-Personalised-Cancer-Medicine.pdf.

Gusev A, Lawrenson K, Lin X, *et al.* (2019). A transcriptome-wide association study of high-grade serous epithelial ovarian cancer identifies new susceptibility genes and splice variants. *Nature Genetics, 51*(5), 815–823. doi:10.1038/s41588-019-0395-x.

Hassen E, Eggert LJT. (2016). Genetic risk and hereditary cancer syndromes. In Yarbro CH, Wujcki D, Holmes GB. (Eds.), *Cancer Nursing: Principles and Practice* (8th ed., pp. 135–168). Burlington, MA: Jones and Bartlett Learning.

Hedditch EL, Gao B, Russell AJ, *et al.* (2014). ABCA transporter gene expression and poor outcome in epithelial ovarian cancer. *Journal of the National Cancer Institute, 106*(7), dju149. doi:10.1093/jnci/dju149.

Lei G, Frommel SC, Oakes CC, *et al.* (2015). BAZ2A (TIP5) is involved in epigenetic alterations in prostate cancer and its overexpression predicts disease recurrence. *Nature Genetics, 47*(1), 22–30.

Lister Hill National Center for Biomedical Communications, U.S. National Library of Medicine, National Institutes of Health, Department of Health, Human Services. (2016). *Help me Understand Genetics.* Bethesda, MD: U.S. National Library of Medicine. Retrieved from https://ghr.nlm.nih.gov/primer.

National Cancer Institute. (2013). *Genetic Testing for Hereditary Cancer Syndromes.* Retrieved from https://www.cancer.gov/about-cancer/causes-prevention/genetics/genetic-testing-fact-sheet.

National Institutes of Health. Genetic conditions: Cancers. *Genetics Home Reference.* Bethesda, MD: U.S. National Library of Medicine.

Perez RE, Shen H, Duan L, *et al.* (2016). Modeling the etiology of p53-mutated cancer cells. *The Journal of Biological Chemistry, 291*(19), 10131–10147. doi:10.1074/jbc.M116.724781.

Robson M, Storm C, Weitzel J, *et al.* (2010). American society of clinical oncology policy statement update: Genetic and genomic testing for cancer susceptibility. *Journal of Clinical Oncology, 28*(5), 893–901.

Samuels Y, Bardelli A, Gartner JJ, *et al.* (2015). *Cancer: Principles and Practice of Oncology* (10th ed., pp. 2–23). Philadelphia: Wolters Kluwer Health/Lippincott Williams & Wilkins.

Waddell N, Pajic M, Patch AM, *et al.* (2015). Whole genomes redefine the mutational landscape of pancreatic cancer. *Nature, 518*(7540), 495–501. doi:10.1038/nature14169.

Wyszynski A, Hong CC, Lam K, *et al.* (2016). An intergenic risk locus containing an enhancer deletion in 2q35 modulates breast cancer risk by deregulating IGFBP5 expression. *Human Molecular Genetics, 25*(17), 3863–3876. doi:10.1093/hmg/ddw223.

Zhao D, Tahaney WM, Mazumdar A, Savage MI, Brown PH. (2017). Molecularly targeted therapies for p53-mutant cancers. *Cellular and Molecular Life Sciences: CMLS, 74*(22), 4171–4187. doi:10.1007/s00018-017-2575-0.

Zhao J, Zhao D, Poage GM, *et al.* (2015). Death-associated protein kinase 1 promotes growth of p53-mutant cancers. *The Journal of Clinical Investigation, 125*(7), 2707–2720. doi:10.1172/JCI70805.

Chapter 3

African Diets Have Lower Cancer Risk

Food plays an important role in the life of every creature on earth. However, what you eat has a tremendous effect on your health. We all have our special meals or diets depending on how they are prepared and their origin. Foods of different origin have different characteristics that make them unique from others. For instance, due to influx of immigrants, America has a rich diversity in food preparation leading to a variety of dishes such as Hawaiian haystack, jambalaya, Yeung Chow fried rice, hamburger, chimichanga, and oysters Rockefeller. Africa has a wide array of cuisines enjoyed across its region with most of them containing very high starch, meat, and spice. Fufu, kenkey, gari, potjiekos, couscous, xalwo, injera, and ful medames are examples of indigenous cuisines enjoyed by most people across the continent, which are mostly high in fiber (Figs. 1–3).

Thanks to medical research, consumers have been made aware of the benefits and consequences of what they eat. There are dozens of reports on the devastating effects of excessive fat and oil, and salt on the body, likewise the health benefits of most nutrients. The latest discovery in cancer medicine is the association of diet to cancer risk. An internationally recognized team of scientists from the

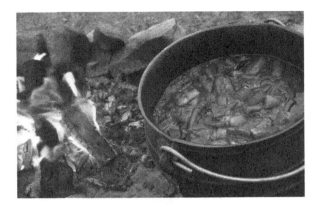

Fig. 1.   Potjie from South Africa

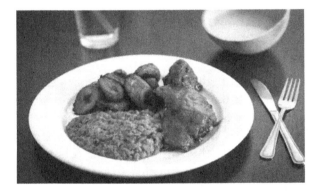

Fig. 2.   Gari and beans (G)b3) from Ghana

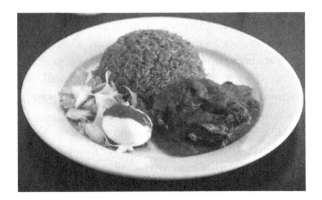

Fig. 3.   Jollof rice from Ghana

University of Pittsburgh and Imperial College London has conducted a well-controlled study on the effects of diets on colon cancer risk for Africans and Americans. Colon cancer is the fourth leading cancer in the world, resulting in about 600,000 deaths each year. This deadly type of cancer is highly seen among African Americans than Africans. In the study, 20 participants each of African Americans and Africans who were on their normal diet were recruited; the bacteria in their colon were also sampled and tested. More than half of the participants from America were seen to have increased inflammation resulting in the formation of polyps — a harmless abnormal growth that can progress to cancer — in their bowel lining. These subjects also had high biomarkers for colon cancer risk while subjects from African had none of these recorded abnormalities.

The scientists swapped the diets of these subjects for two weeks and the findings were incredible. A marked decrease in polyps formation and biomarkers for cancer risk was recorded for the subjects from America. However, the subjects from Africa who initially had no abnormalities were seen to develop increased inflammation leading to polyps formation with increased biomarkers for colon cancer risk. The investigators have attributed these tremendous colon changes to the food constituents and microbiome — bacteria in the gut. This relation is not new to cancer research, however. The significant changes realized in that shortest possible time are something remarkable and surprising, as mentioned by Prof. Jeremy Nicholson, Department of Surgery and Cancer at the Imperial College London (Fig. 4).

Comparatively, American diets contain higher fat, protein, and lower amount of fiber than that of African origin. Dietary fibers have been shown to have protective effects against colorectal cancers, mainly due to its fermentation to butyrate by the gut bacteria. According to Bultman SJ of Lineberger Comprehensive Cancer Centre, University of North Carolina, moderate fiber leads to the formation of low to moderate levels of butyrate that serves as a food source for the colonocytes — cells of the colon. Butyrate undergoes beta-oxidation in mitochondria to generate about 70% of energy for the normal colonocytes. A very high amount of dietary fiber therefore leads to the accumulation of unmetabolized butyrate in the cell

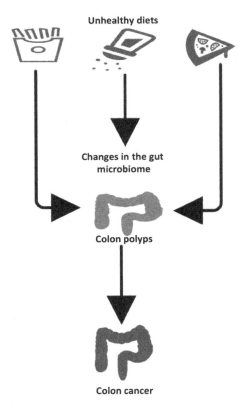

Fig. 4.   Highly refined foods change the microbe composition in our intestines, leading to an increase in cancer risk

nucleus, acting as histone deacetylase inhibitor to inhibit cell prolif-eration and induce apoptosis. These cumulative effects contribute to the decreased levels of polyps formation and biomarkers for colon cancer risk. The protective effect of dietary-related butyrate has also been reported by McIntyre A, Department of Medicine at the University of Melbourne and Julia Wong, Clinical Nutrition and Risk Factor Modification at the St. Michael's Hospital, Toronto.

Beside butyrate, a Japanese scientist called Ohsawa Ikuroh from Nippon Medical School has reported on the potential protective antioxidant effects of hydrogen — a by-product of fiber metabolism — against colorectal cancer. On the other hand, increased dietary fat may result in increased unabsorbed lipid metabolites — after gut bacteria metabolism — which create lethal injuries on the colon mucosa causing reactive hyperproliferation. Some absorbed lipid metabolites could also transform into active biological products that could be a potential cancer-causing agent.

The gut microbiome therefore plays a key role in maintaining the integrity of the colon mucosa. The diets we eat, however, affect their distribution and hence a change in the mucosa. Gut microbiome could therefore be explored for therapeutic prospects not only for cancer but for other inflammatory-related diseases. Further investigation on butyrate should be encouraged to gain in-depth knowledge in its anticancer properties and other possible health benefits.

Most diets of African origin have very low lactose but high calcium components that are key determinants of risk factors for ovarian cancer development in African Americans. In the *American Journal of Clinical Nutrition*, a similar observation was demonstrated where high lactose but low calcium consumptions were associated with the aggressive form of prostate cancer. In addition, Western diets unlike the African diets are pro-inflammatory, which provide the congenial environment for tumor growth and immune cell suppression. Switching of diet to African meals has been demonstrated to show reduction in polyps formation, a condition that can progress over time to colon cancer.

Other than the food differences, the gut microbiota differences between races or ethnic groups could also contribute massively to tumor growth. Thus, an African American's gut microbiota might respond differently to Western diets, creating suitable conditions for cancer development. The reverse could also be true in the case of Caucasians or Asian. In a study published in the *British Journal of Nutrition*, black South African women were advised to eat more fruits and vegetables that reduce their risk of breast cancer. Beside the nutritional values in vegetables and fruits that contribute to the overall good health of the consumer, the gut microbiota of these ethnic groups might effectively metabolize the nutrients into products that can provide protection against tumor compared with other races. Also, other ethnic groups could be able to handle the effects of red meat as well as high energy foods compared with African women due to differences in gut microbiota.

After these findings, one will be tempted to ask the state of the colons of most African Americans who have lived in America for more than 10 years. Obviously, their colon mucosa will have more polyps compared to that of their African counterparts. This should serve as a warning to Africans living a Westernized life regardless of their country of residence. This work is not about American foods, but rather, eating food rich in fiber and low fat. The progressive Westernization of Africans could therefore mean progressive cancer development. It is not always about what you eat, rather, what you feed the gut microbiome with. The power lies in your hands to embrace cancer or life. Stay true to African diets.

The chemopreventive nature of meals from Africa has nothing to do with the land of Africa or how these meals come about but rather their nutritional components. Meals from Africa are rich in dietary fibers, calcium, and other chemopreventive nutrients, unlike the Western diets which are mostly rich in lactose and nutrients that support cancer growth. The location is likely not to play any role in this association and does not suggest that people should travel to Africa in order to experience these health benefits. Changing the nutrient composition in the Western diets could provide similar chemopreventive benefits to consumers. It is worth knowing that other foods from Asia have nutrient composition similar to that of Africa and hence are likely to possess these health benefits. Although the nutrient composition is crucial, the gut microbiota could also play a critical role in the metabolism of these nutrients that could either prevent or support tumor growth. It is yet to be demonstrated if the gut microbiota composition differences between Africans and Caucasians play a role in the nutritional benefits from diets. Should there be a difference, microbiota transplant could be exploited as an alternative therapeutic approach. As the old saying goes, "you are what you eat." Thus, how healthy you are is largely dependent on how healthy your food is. Having the right composition of food could be a cheaper way of staying away from the doctor and other health complications.

Bibliography

Brasky TM, Sponholtz TR, Palmer JR, Rosenberg L, Ruiz-Narváez EA, Wise LA. (2016). Associations of dietary long-chain ω-3 polyunsaturated fatty acids and fish consumption with endometrial cancer risk in the black women's health study. *American Journal of Epidemiology, 183*(3), 199–209. doi:10.1093/aje/kwv231.

Bultman SJ. (2016). Butyrate consumption of differentiated colonocytes in the upper crypt promotes homeostatic proliferation of stem and progenitor cells near the crypt base. *Translational Cancer Research, 5,* S526–S528. doi:10.21037/tcr.2016.08.36.

Bultman SJ. (2017). Interplay between diet, gut microbiota, epigenetic events, and colorectal cancer. *Molecular Nutrition & Food Research, 61*(1). doi:10.1002/mnfr.201500902.

Feng YL, Shu L, Zheng PF, *et al.* (2016). Dietary patterns and colorectal cancer risk: A meta-analysis. *European Cancer Prevention Organisation, 26*(3), 201–211. doi:10.1097/CEJ.0000000000000245.

Jacobs I, Taljaard-Krugell C, Ricci C, *et al.* (2019). Dietary intake and breast cancer risk in black South African women: The South African breast cancer study. *The British Journal of Nutrition, 121*(5), 591–600. doi:10.1017/S0007114518003744.

McIntyre A, Gibson PR, Young GP. (1993). Butyrate production from dietary fibre and protection against large bowel cancer in a rat model. *Gut, 34*(3), 386–391. doi:10.1136/gut.34.3.386.

Ohsawa I, Ishikawa M, Takahashi K, *et al.* (2007). Hydrogen acts as a therapeutic antioxidant by selectively reducing cytotoxic oxygen radicals. *Nature Medicine, 13,* 688–694. doi:10.1038/nm1577.

O'Keefe SJD, Li JV, Lahti L, *et al.* (2015). Fat, fibre and cancer risk in African Americans and rural Africans. *Nature Communications, 6,* 6342. doi:10.1038/ncomms7342.

Peres LC, Bandera EV, Qin B, *et al.* (2017). Dietary inflammatory index and risk of epithelial ovarian cancer in African American women. *International Journal of Cancer, 140*(3), 535–543. doi:10.1002/ijc.30467

Qin B, Moorman PG, Alberg AJ, *et al.* (2016). Dairy, calcium, vitamin D and ovarian cancer risk in African-American women. *British Journal of Cancer, 115*(9), 1122–1130. doi:10.1038/bjc.2016.289.

Steck SE, Omofuma OO, Su LJ, *et al.* (2018). Calcium, magnesium, and whole-milk intakes and high-aggressive prostate cancer in the North

Carolina-Louisiana Prostate Cancer Project (PCaP). *American Society for Clinical Nutrition, 107*(5), 799–807. doi:10.1093/ajcn/nqy037.

Theodoratou E, Timofeeva M, Li X, Meng X, Ioannidis J. (2017). Nature, nurture, and cancer risks: Genetic and nutritional contributions to cancer. *Annual Review of Nutrition, 37,* 293–320. doi:10.1146/annurev-nutr-071715-051004.

Turner ND, Lloyd SK. (2017). Association between red meat consumption and colon cancer: A systematic review of experimental results. *Experimental Biology and Medicine, 242*(8), 813–839. doi:10.1177/1535370217693117.

Zheng J, Guinter MA, Merchant AT, *et al.* (2017). Dietary patterns and risk of pancreatic cancer: A systematic review. *Nutrition Reviews, 75*(11), 883–908. doi:10.1093/nutrit/nux038.

Zitvogel L, Pietrocola F, Kroemer G. (2017). Nutrition, inflammation and cancer. *Nature Immunology, 18,* 843–850. doi:10.1038/ni.3754.

Chapter 4

Alcohol Intake: A Simple Way to the Cancer Kingdom

Alcohol has become a commodity that has gained popularity in every corner of the world. With a growing demand for alcoholic beverages, brewery companies have multiplied over the past two decades to meet demands. Alcohol is basically produced when yeasts act on sugars or starch by a process called fermentation. Alcohol is the common name for ethanol and aside beverages, it is also found in medicines, perfumes, essential oils, mouthwash, and other household products. People have attributed their consumption of alcohol to religious beliefs, cultural, medical reasons, and emotional situations, among others. The question is, are these people aware that alcoholic beverages are considered as group 1 carcinogen — a substance that has the ability to cause cancer — by the International Agency for Research on Cancer (IARC)? I guess no. Alcohol beverage consumption has been reported to cause the following cancers: esophageal, oral cavity, pharynx, larynx, colorectal, female breast, and probably prostate cancer according to IARC.

There have been extensive studies across the globe that provide some level of evidence to confirm the alcohol–cancer association. Boffetta Paolo has earlier recorded in a study that 3.6% of all cancer

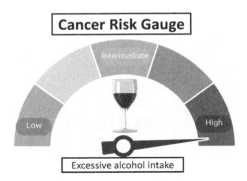

Fig. 1. Excessive intake of alcohol increases cancer risk

cases and 3.5% of all cancer deaths are related to alcohol intake. In 2009, ABC News 24 reported that 21,000 Australians die from alcohol-related cancer each year in Australia. The BBC News also reported in 2011 that alcohol intake leads to 1 in 10 cancers in men and 1 in 33 cancers in women. A 2011 study by Parkin DM and Cancer Research UK in the United Kingdom has shown 12,000 alcohol-related cancer cases per year with bowel cancer accounting for the highest (Fig. 1).

With regards to how alcohol consumption increases the risk of cancer, researchers have identified several mechanisms to explain this association. According to Cancer Research UK, alcohol when consumed is metabolized to acetaldehyde, which is a known human carcinogen; acetaldehyde can cause damage to the DNA and proteins that could eventually lead to cancer. Apart from alcohol metabolism in the liver, other bacteria in the mouth and gut linings could metabolize alcohol into acetaldehyde, therefore increasing the risk of cancer in the mouth and gut. Alcohol metabolism could also generate free radicals such as reactive oxygen species (ROS) that can damage the DNA, protein, and other essential lipids. Acetaldehyde also has the ability to increase the growth of liver cells abnormally, which could ultimately lead to cancer. Alcohol can also influence the increased production of hormones such as estrogen that serves as a chemical messenger to instruct the division of cells. High blood levels of estrogen are associated with increased risk of breast cancer. During the fermentation and production process, carcinogenic substances such as phenols, nitrosamines, hydrocarbons, and asbestos fibers contaminate the alcohol, thereby further increasing the cancer risk.

The question that people normally ask is "what is the safe dose of alcohol one needs to consume to be healthy"? In most alcohol beverage commercials, customers are encouraged to drink responsibly; however, when it comes to cancer, there is nothing like a safe dose of alcohol. This is confirmed in the 2014 World Cancer Report issued by the IARC. The risk is dose-dependent; thus, the higher the consumption of alcohol, the higher your cancer risk. In two meta-analyses conducted by Tramacere and Bagnardi — these two experts conducted separate studies — they concluded that one alcohol drink a day can increase cancer risk. In Bagnardi's meta-analysis, it was shown that light drinkers have a high risk of oropharyngeal cancer, esophageal squamous cell carcinoma, and female breast cancer than nondrinkers. I, however, see a caveat in this study since there is a high probability that the light drinkers could have underestimated their alcohol intake. This can affect the entire finding and not give a true reflection on the light alcohol intake/cancer risk association. Notwithstanding, there is lots of scientific evidence to show that cancer risk is dose-dependent (Fig. 2).

A little amount of alcohol has been revealed to offer some level of cardiac protection for people at risk of heart diseases.

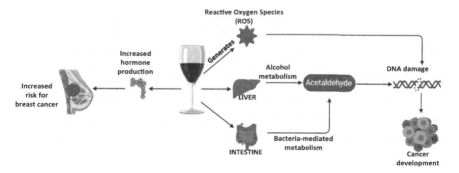

Fig. 2. Excessive alcohol intake regulates multiple pathways that promote the development of cancer

However, increasing the amount of alcohol with the intention of improving health has no correlation. Rather, you increase your risk of other health complications such as stroke, hypertension, and cancer. *"Moderate drinking — between 1 and 2 units a day — has been shown to offer some protection against heart disease. However, this should not be seen by people as a green light to start drinking — as there are better ways to protect your heart. Eating a sensible diet, exercising regularly and stopping smoking are all much better ways to keep your heart healthy,"* said Dr. Mike Knapton, Associate Medical Director, British Heart Foundation.

Another controversy is with red wine. Many alcohol lovers hide behind the health benefits of red wine and abuse their alcohol intake. Dr. Patel KR of the Department of Cancer Studies and Molecular Medicine, University of Leicester, has found substances like resveratrol in red wine that possesses anticancer properties. However, clinical trials at the Department of Dermatology, College of Physicians and Surgeons, Columbia University, did not provide any evidence that resveratrol could be used in cancer treatment or prevention. Red wine abusers should have this in mind when increasing their intake of red wine thinking it is improving their health.

Excessive alcohol intake could lead to increased metabolites that have the ability to suppress immune cell functions. With immune suppression, cancers have the upper hand to grow, multiply, and spread to other locations — conditions that complicate treatment and shorten patients' survival. Thus, reduced or eliminating alcohol consumption could help boost the immune system for effective immune-surveillance. There have also been reports where alcohol consumption contraindicates cancer treatments. In prostate cancer patients, alcohol consumption inhibits the therapeutic effects of 5α-reductase inhibitors. This contributes to increased cancer aggressiveness and poor patient survival. It's therefore recommendable that patients avoid alcohol intake to achieve full therapeutic success when undergoing treatments. This might not pertain to only prostate cancer patients but could also be extended to other types of cancer patients.

With the increasing cancer mortality, people should make conscious efforts to abhor lifestyles that can increase their risk of cancer. The devastating effects of alcohol intake far outweigh its health benefits, hence care should be taken when patronizing alcohol-serving establishments. Always have in mind that the little alcohol you consume has its corresponding cancer risk and the higher the intake, the higher the risk. The effects are even more damaging when alcohol usage is combined with smoking. It has been reported that alcohol increases the rate at which the chemicals in the cigarette are assimilated into the blood. Also, the metabolites from alcohol could combine with those from tobacco to cause more damaging effects. It is worth understanding that cancer risk increases with increase in alcohol consumption and the earlier this lifestyle is checked, the better.

Bibliography

Ahmad Kiadaliri A, Jarl J, Gavriilidis G, Gerdtham UG. (2013). Alcohol drinking cessation and the risk of laryngeal and pharyngeal cancers: A systematic review and meta-analysis. *PLoS One, 8*(3), e58158.

Baan R, Straif K, Grosse Y, *et al.* (2007). Carcinogenicity of alcoholic beverages. *The Lancet Oncology, 8,* 292–293. doi:10.1016/S1470-2045 (07)70099-2.

Bagnardi V, Rota M, Botteri E, *et al.* (2015). Alcohol consumption and site-specific cancer risk: A comprehensive dose-response meta-analysis. *British Journal of Cancer, 112*(3), 580–593. doi:10.1038/bjc.2014.579.

Bemis DL, Katz AE, Buttyan R. (2006). Clinical trials of natural products as chemopreventive agents for prostate cancer. *Expert Opinion on InvestigationalDrugs, 15*(10),1191–1200.doi:10.1517/13543784.15.10.1191

Boffetta P, Hashibe M. (2006). Alcohol and cancer. *The Lancet Oncology, 7,* 149–156. doi:10.1016/S1470-2045(06)70577-0.

Cao Y, Willett WC, Rimm EB, Stampfer MJ, Giovannucci EL. (2015). Light to moderate intake of alcohol, drinking patterns, and risk of cancer: Results from two prospective US cohort studies. *BMJ, 351,* h4238.

Chao C, Haque R, Caan BJ, Poon KY, Tseng HF, Quinn VP. (2010). Red wine consumption not associated with reduced risk of colorectal cancer. *Nutrition and Cancer, 62*(6), 849–855.

Druesne-Pecollo N, Tehard B, Mallet Y, *et al.* (2009). Alcohol and genetic polymorphisms: Effect on risk of alcohol-related cancer. *Lancet Oncology, 10*(2), 173–180.

Fedirko V, Tramacere I, Bagnardi V, *et al.* (2011). Alcohol drinking and colorectal cancer risk: An overall and dose–response meta-analysis of published studies. *Annals of Oncology, 22*(9), 1958–1972. doi:10.1093/annonc/mdq653.

GBD 2016 Alcohol Collaborators. (2018). Alcohol use and burden for 195 countries and territories, 1990–2016: A systematic analysis for the Global Burden of Disease Study 2016. *Lancet, 392*(10152), 1015–1035. doi:10.1016/S0140-6736(18)31310-2.

Gescher A, Steward WP, Brown K. (2013). Resveratrol in the management of human cancer: How strong is the clinical evidence? *Annals of the New York Academy of Sciences, 1290*, 12–20.

Gomella L. (2014). Alcohol, cancer and 5α-reductase inhibitors — Is there a link? *Nature Reviews: Urology, 11*, 253–254. doi:10.1038/nrurol.2014.90

https://www.bbc.com/news/av/health-13009113/alcohol-can-increase-cancer-risk.

https://www.telegraph.co.uk/science/2018/01/03/drinking-alcohol-raises-risk-cancer-snapping-dna-scientists/.

IARC Monographs on the Evaluation of Carcinogenic Risks to Humans. (1988). *Alcohol drinking* (Vol. 44). Lyon: International Agency for Research on Cancer.

International Agency for Research on Cancer, World Health Organisation (WHO). (October 24, 2019). Retrieved from https://monographs.iarc.fr/list-of-classifications.

Pandeya N, Williams G, Green AC, Webb PM, Whiteman DC, Australian Cancer Study. (2009). Alcohol consumption and the risks of adenocarcinoma and squamous cell carcinoma of the esophagus. *Gastroenterology, 136*(4), 1215–1224, e1–2. doi:10.1053/j.gastro.2008.12.052.

Parkin DM. (2011). Cancers attributable to consumption of alcohol in the UK in 2010. *British Journal of Cancer, 105*(Suppl. 2), S14–S18. doi:10.1038/bjc.2011.476.

Patel KR, Brown VA, Jones DJ, *et al.* (2010). Clinical pharmacology of resveratrol and its metabolites in colorectal cancer patients. *Cancer Research, 70*(19), 7392–7399.

Rehm J, Patra J, Popova S. (2007). Alcohol drinking cessation and its effect on esophageal and head and neck cancers: A pooled analysis. *International Journal of Cancer, 121*(5), 1132–1137.

Stornetta A, Guidolin V, Balbo S. (2018). Alcohol-derived acetaldehyde exposure in the oral cavity. *Cancers, 10*(1), pii: E20.

Turati F, Garavello W, Tramacere I, *et al.* (2013). A meta-analysis of alcohol drinking and oral and pharyngeal cancers: Results from subgroup analyses. *Alcohol and Alcoholism, 48*(1), 107–118.

Ugai T, Kelemen LE, Mizuno M, *et al.* (2018). Ovarian cancer risk, ALDH2 polymorphism and alcohol drinking: Asian data from the Ovarian Cancer Association Consortium. *Cancer Science, 109*(2), 435–445. doi:10.1111/cas.13470.

Vartolomei MD, Kimura S, Ferro M, *et al.* (2018). The impact of moderate wine consumption on the risk of developing prostate cancer. *Clinical Epidemiology, 10*, 431–444.

Wang Z, Fan J, Liu M, *et al.* (2013). Nutraceuticals for prostate cancer chemoprevention: From molecular mechanisms to clinical application. *Expert Opinion on Investigational Drugs, 22*(12), 1613–1626.

White AJ, DeRoo LA, Weinberg CR, Sandler DP. (2017). Lifetime alcohol intake, binge drinking behaviors, and breast cancer risk. *American Journal of Epidemiology, 186*(5), 541–549.

Chapter 5

Caution to Egg Lovers

Eggs are body-building foods that contain essential nutrients such as vitamin A, D, iron, choline, linoleic acid, among others. These nutrients are necessary for the perfect functioning of the human system. Despite these wonderful body-building functions, eggs have also been implicated in several cardiovascular disorders — although a weak link has been established. An emerging health complication of eggs is their association to cancer risk.

A multisite case-control study in Uruguay led by Aune Dagfinn and published in the *Asian Pacific Journal of Cancer Prevention* has revealed an association between higher intake of eggs and increased risk of several cancers at nine different organ sites including the breast, colon, lung, prostate, bladder, and esophagus. The author and colleagues during this study took into consideration the adjustment of other parameters that can influence the outcome of the results such as age, sex, smoking, alcohol intake, fruits intake, body mass index (BMI), and fatty food/meat intake.

A twofold increase in prostate cancer risk has also been revealed in a study conducted by researchers from Harvard University, the University of California in San Francisco, and the Women's Hospital in the United States. An 81% high risk of lethal prostate cancer was reported in men who ate an average of 2.5 or more eggs per week as compared to those who had only less than half an egg per week. Smoking habits, age, sex, BMI, and other confounding factors of the 27,607 subjects were controlled.

At the School of Population Health, University of Queensland Medical School, Australia, Sandi Pirozzo has shown a similar link where high intake of eggs resulted in increased ovarian cancer risk.

Increased cholesterol associated with egg consumption was thought to be the reason for the increased cancer risk; however, this assertion has been flawed by many findings including that of Sandi Pirozzo of the University of Queensland Medical School. Studies have shown that up to one egg a day is unlikely to cause increase in cardiovascular-related disorders in healthy individuals.

Race is also a key player in the association between cancer risk and egg consumption. In the *Journal of Breast Cancer*, the authors demonstrated a significant positive association between egg consumption and breast cancer among Europeans and Asians but not Americans. Postmenopausal populations were also at higher risk compared with premenopausal women. In this same study, subjects who consumed more than two eggs per week were significantly associated with increased risk of breast cancer compared with those who ate less. In another study, a positive dose–response association was observed between excessive egg consumption (greater than five eggs per week) and gastrointestinal cancers especially with colon cancers. Although egg consumption might predispose a person to cancer development, the amount of consumption and ethnicity might play a huge role in the process. Other studies have also shown that cancer risk is significantly increased by the consumption of fried eggs compared with other forms. Thus, the way an egg is prepared before

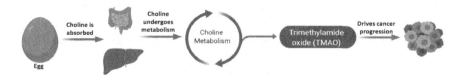

Fig. 1.   Choline from eggs serves as a source of fuel that is capable of driving cancer growth

consumption could also influence its association with cancer risk. This observation was realized when increased fried egg consumption but not other forms was significantly associated with bladder cancer.

Although egg consumption is highly associated with cancer risk, other studies have shown contrary results. In a study published in the *Journal of Nutrition and Cancer*, the authors demonstrated that people who consumed two eggs per week are 62% less likely to develop glioma compared with those who ate less. Gliomas are types of cancers that occur in the brain and spinal cords. These tumors are very aggressive and usually result in poor prognosis. Thus, depending on the amount taken, egg consumption could either be beneficial or detrimental to the consumer. Regardless, the tumor-promoting effects outweigh the tumor protection properties of eggs.

Eggs are highly concentrated with choline that has been shown to increase the risk of cancer initiation, spread and lethality (Fig. 1); increase in choline is associated with 70% increased risk of prostate cancer. In healthy cells, oxygen and citrate serve as the main raw materials for energy production. However, in cancer cells, choline is used to generate energy for the growth of malignant cells. The choline is converted to trimethylamide oxide (TMAO) in the gut and liver that leads to inflammation and ultimately carcinogenesis.

Regardless of the fact that choline is a known contributing factor of several cancers, other studies have reported its health benefits such as maintaining the integrity of cell membrane and the synthesis of neurotransmitter for the effective functioning of coordination signals. It is therefore imperative for researchers to determine the dietary reference intake (DRI) to ensure the safe dose of choline. Also, there is the need for further investigation on the molecular and cellular mechanisms of choline in carcinogenesis to identify promising therapeutic targets. A clear understanding of the function of choline will be beneficial in designing potential treatment modalities for cancer patients. Choline might not be the only cancer-promoting substance in eggs, hence more studies are needed to investigate the potential of other substances contained in eggs. This does not in any way rule out the health benefits obtained from eggs. Taking eggs in moderate amount is recommended and could provide the necessary health benefit needed without any adverse effects.

Individuals should exercise caution not to abuse the consumption of eggs in their quest to achieving their full health benefits, since growing evidence has shown the association between higher egg intake and increased cancer risk.

Bibliography

Aminianfar A, Fallah-Moshkani R, Salari-Moghaddam A, Saneei P, Larijani B, Esmaillzadeh A. (2019). Egg consumption and risk of upper aerodigestive tract cancers: A systematic review and meta-analysis of observational studies. *Advances in Nutrition, 10*(4), 660–672.

Aminianfar A, Shayanfar M, Mohammad-Shirazi M, Sharifi G, Esmaillzadeh A. (2019). Egg consumption in relation to glioma: A case-control study. *Nutrition and Cancer, 71*(1), 41–49. doi:10.1080/016 35581.2018.1540712.

Aune D, De Stefani E, Ronco AL, *et al.* (2009). Egg consumption and the risk of cancer: A multisite case-control study in Uruguay. *Asian Pacific Journal of Cancer Prevention: APJCP, 10*(5), 869–876.

Fang D, Tan F, Wang C, Zhu X, Xie L. (2012). Egg intake and bladder cancer risk: A meta-analysis. *Experimental and Therapeutic Medicine, 4*(5), 906–912. doi:10.3892/etm.2012.671.

Keum N, Lee D, Marchand N, *et al.* (2015). Egg intake and cancers of the breast, ovary and prostate: A dose–response meta-analysis of prospective observational studies. *British Journal of Nutrition, 114*(7), 1099–1107. doi:10.1017/S0007114515002135.

Larsson SC, Håkanson N, Permert J, Wolk A. (2006). Meat, fish, poultry and egg consumption in relation to risk of pancreatic cancer: A prospective study. *International Journal of Cancer, 118*(11), 2866–2870.

Li F, Zhou Y, Hu RT, *et al.* (2013). Egg consumption and risk of bladder cancer: A meta-analysis. *Nutrition and Cancer, 65*(4), 538–546. doi:10.10 80/01635581.2013.770041.

Luo H, Sun P, He S, Guo S, Guo Y. (2019). A meta-analysis of the association between poultry and egg consumption and the risk of brain cancer. *Cellular and Molecular Biology, 65*(1), 14–18.

Pirozzo S, Purdie D, Kuiper-Linley M, *et al.* (2002). Ovarian cancer, cholesterol, and eggs: A case-control analysis. *Cancer Epidemiology Biomarkers and Prevention, 11*(101), 1112–1114.

Richman EL, Kenfield SA, Stampfer MJ, Giovannucci EL, Chan JM. (2011). Egg, red meat, and poultry intake and risk of lethal prostate cancer in the prostate-specific antigen-era: Incidence and survival. *Cancer Prevention Research (Philadelphia, PA.), 4*(12), 2110–2121. doi:10.1158/1940-6207. CAPR-11-0354.

Si R, Qu K, Jiang Z, Yang X, Gao P. (2014). Egg consumption and breast cancer risk: A meta-analysis. *Breast Cancer, 21*(3), 251–261. doi:10.1007/s12282-014-0519-1.

Tse G, Eslick GD. (2014). Egg consumption and risk of GI neoplasms: Dose-response meta-analysis and systematic review. *European Journal of Nutrition, 53*(7), 1581–1590.

Zeng ST, Guo L, Liu SK, *et al.* (2015). Egg consumption is associated with increased risk of ovarian cancer: Evidence from a meta-analysis of observational studies. *Clinical Nutrition, 34*(4), 635–641.

Zhang C, Ho SC, Chen Y, Lin FY, Fu JH, Cheng SZ. (2009). Meat and egg consumption and risk of breast cancer among Chinese women. *Cancer Causes & Control, 20*, 1845–1853. doi:10.1007/s10552-009-9377-0.

Chapter 6

Coffee Protects Against Cancer Risk and Recurrence

There is growing evidence of how diets and lifestyles influence cancer risk, survival, and treatment. It is much speculated that coffee consumption causes serious health complications without any scientific proof. Recent studies have refuted these rumors and rather hailed coffee as a promising therapeutic agent to increase the survival rate of cancer patients (Fig. 1).

The American Association for Cancer Research has reported a 39% decrease in oral and head cancer recurrence in patients who consumed four cups of coffee daily. A 60% decrease in prostate cancer risk was also reported in men who consumed six cups of coffee daily.

Crystal Holick and colleagues at the University of Harvard, United States, have revealed a 40% decrease in brain cancer risk in people who consume five cups of coffee daily. These results come as great news to the cancer research community since brain cancer is one of the deadliest cancers to treat and manage. In recent studies, coffee intake has been significantly associated with lower risk of developing breast cancer as well as other gynecological cancers.

Another study on the association of coffee consumption and reduced cancer risk has been documented in the *Journal of Clinical*

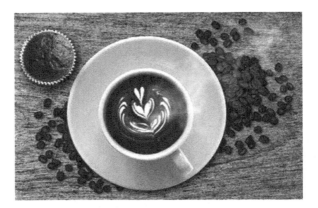

Fig. 1.   Coffee

Oncology by a group of researchers from the Dana-Farber Cancer Institute. Their findings revealed that frequent consumption of caffeinated coffee provided a 42% less recurrence in stage 3 colon cancer patients while a 33% improved survival was also achieved. Similar improved survival rates have been reported in liver, endometrial, lung, and skin cancer patients (Fig. 2).

A study on epithelial ovarian cancer reported that considerate intake of coffee or caffeine resulted in no significant susceptibility to ovarian cancer; however, it might offer some level of protection against this cancer. This adds up to an array of studies that have demonstrated that coffee intake is significantly associated with reduced incidences of cancer and other fatal health conditions. In an eight population-based cohort study in Japan, researchers found that consuming up to five cups of coffee per day might offer health benefits against mortality resulting from major causes. In a Swedish population study, the authors also found that coffee intake is significantly associated with reduced risk of gall bladder cancer. A reduced prostate cancer risk was also observed with coffee intake in a meta-analysis of prospective cohort studies. In Norwegian women, a modest reduction in cancer risk was demonstrated with coffee intake. In a study conducted with subjects from Northern Israel, people who consumed more coffee had 26% lower odds of developing colorectal cancers compared with people who did not drink

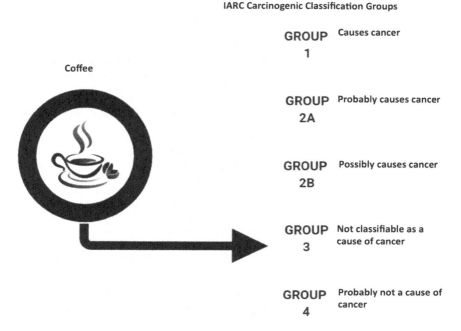

Fig. 2. Coffee is not classifiable as a cancer-causing agent

coffee. This association was more significant with increase in the number of cups taken per week. Specifically, greater than 2.5 cups a week provide significant protection against colon and rectal cancers. A Japanese study has further demonstrated that not only does coffee consumption reduce the risk of colorectal cancers but also help prevent cancers that affect the tail end of the intestines called distal colon cancer.

In a European-based investigation published in the *International Journal of Cancer*, antitumor protection ability of Italian-style coffee was studied. At the epidemiological level, people who consumed more than three cups of Italian-style coffee per day had 53% lower risk of prostate cancer compared with those who consumed no to fewer cups of coffee. At the cellular level, human prostate cancer cell lines were treated with caffeine to demonstrate if coffee truly exerts antitumor properties. It was demonstrated that caffeine inhibited the ability of the prostate cancer cell lines to proliferate (grow) and metastasize (move to other sites of the body).

The findings above strongly demonstrate that coffee consumption offers cancer protection and could be beneficial to healthy people. This protection is regardless of race and ethnicity of the consumer as these studies involve participants from America, Asia, Africa, and Europe. Also, the protection was not tied to a particular brand of coffee. Thus, every coffee regardless of the origin has the capacity to provide some level of health benefits. Although these findings are promising and interesting, there are limitations that need to be addressed. Confounding factors such as age, sex, and genes should be investigated to see how they influence coffee responses. In a European cohort study, tea but not coffee was shown to be involved in the epigenetic regulation of DNA, which could influence cancer growth. We have yet to also demonstrate if lifestyles such as smoking, unhealthy eating, inactivity, and drugs affect the health benefits of coffee. To date, there is no medically accepted dose of coffee recommended to be used worldwide; thus, consumption rate differs from one region to another. Also, the climate might influence the consumption of coffee as people living in colder regions such as Canada and the Scandinavian countries are likely to consume more coffee. People in the tropics or areas with hot weathers are likely to go for cold drinks rather than a hot coffee. Investigating some of these discrepancies could help strengthen the association between coffee consumption and cancer risks (Fig. 3).

One area of research worth investing is to examine if coffee contraindicates treatment effects in cancer patients. Knowledge from such findings could help both cancer patients and clinicians in treatment monitoring and management. Such research themes will involve human cancer cell lines, animal (mouse) model as well as patient studies. It is too early for clinicians to prescribe coffee for cancer patients since more research is needed to establish this association. The ability of coffee consumption to increase cancer patient survival comes as welcoming news to both patients and researchers.

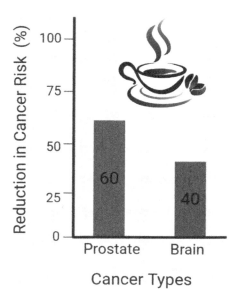

Fig. 3. Coffee intake is significantly associated with reduced risk of prostate and brain cancers

This should be an inspiration for other researchers to investigate the exact mechanism coffee takes to deliver such anticancer benefits. Earlier reports have attributed the anticancer property to biologically active components like antioxidants and minerals found in coffee. Notwithstanding, the cellular and molecular detailing of the anticancer properties of coffee needs to be documented to support its clinical use. Also, the addition of sugar, milk, or cream could either reduce or nullify the health benefits of coffee, hence care should be taken in order to achieve the full health benefits of coffee.

Coffee does not prevent cancer; these studies only show a link of improved survival and decreased cancer risk. Care must be taken not to abuse coffee consumption in your attempt to achieving better health since too much of everything is bad. The key lies in the moderate consumption of coffee while reducing milk and sugar additions.

Bibliography

Abe SK, Saito E, Sawada N, *et al.* (2019). Coffee consumption and mortality in Japanese men and women: A pooled analysis of eight population-based cohort studies in Japan (Japan Cohort Consortium). *Preventive Medicine, 123,* 270–277.

Björner S, Rosendahl AH, Tryggvadottir H, *et al.* (2018). Coffee is associated with lower breast tumor insulin-like growth factor receptor 1 levels in normal-weight patients and improved prognosis following tamoxifen or radiotherapy treatment. *Frontiers in Endocrinology, 9,* 306. doi:10.3389/fendo.2018.00306.

Cao S, Liu L, Yin X, Wang Y, Liu J, Lu Z. (2014). Coffee consumption and risk of prostate cancer: A meta-analysis of prospective cohort studies. *Carcinogenesis, 35*(2), 256–261.

Crippa A, Discacciati A, Larsson SC, Wolk A, Orsini N. (2014). Coffee consumption and mortality from all causes, cardiovascular disease, and cancer: A dose-response meta-analysis. *American Journal of Epidemiology, 180*(8), 763–775.

Ek WE, Tobi EW, Ahsan M, *et al.* (2017). Tea and coffee consumption in relation to DNA methylation in four European cohorts. *Human Molecular Genetics, 26*(16), 3221–3231. doi:10.1093/hmg/ddx194.

Gapstur SM, Anderson RL, Campbell PT, *et al.* (2017). Associations of coffee drinking and cancer mortality in the cancer prevention study-II. *Cancer Epidemiology Biomarkers and Prevention, 26*(10), 1477–1486.

Guercio BJ, Sato K, Niedzwiecki D, *et al.* (2015). Coffee intake, recurrence, and mortality in stage III colon cancer: Results from CALGB 89803 (alliance). *Journal of Clinical Oncology: Official Journal of the American Society of Clinical Oncology, 33*(31), 3598–3607. doi:10.1200/JCO.2015.61.5062.

Holick CN, Smith SG, Giovannucci E, Michaud DS. (2010). Coffee, tea, caffeine intake, and risk of adult glioma in three prospective cohort studies. *Cancer Epidemiology, Biomarkers & Prevention: A Publication of the American Association for Cancer Research, Cosponsored by the American Society of Preventive Oncology, 19*(1), 39–47. doi:10.1158/1055-9965. EPI-09-0732.

Lafranconi A, Micek A, De Paoli P, *et al.* (2018). Coffee intake decreases risk of postmenopausal breast cancer: A dose-response meta-analysis on prospective cohort studies. *Nutrients, 10*(2), 112. doi:10.3390/nu10020112.

Larsson SC, Giovannucci EL, Wolk A. (2017). Coffee consumption and risk of gallbladder cancer in a prospective study. *Journal of the National Cancer Institute, 109*(3), 1–3. doi:10.1093/jnci/djw237.

Lu Y, Zhai L, Zeng J, *et al.* (2014). Coffee consumption and prostate cancer risk: An updated meta-analysis. *Cancer Causes & Control, 25*(5), 591–604.

Lukic M, Licaj I, Lund E, Skeie G, Weiderpass E, Braaten T. (2016). Coffee consumption and the risk of cancer in the Norwegian Women and Cancer (NOWAC) Study. *European Journal of Epidemiology, 31*(9), 905–916. doi:10.1007/s10654-016-0142-x.

Nakagawa-Senda H, Ito H, Hosono S, Oze I, Tanaka H, Matsuo K. (2017). Coffee consumption and the risk of colorectal cancer by anatomical subsite in Japan: Results from the HERPACC studies. *International Journal of Cancer, 141*(2), 298–308. doi:10.1002/ijc.30746.

Ong JS, Hwang LD, Cuellar-Partida G, *et al.* (2018). Assessment of moderate coffee consumption and risk of epithelial ovarian cancer: A Mendelian randomization study. *International Journal of Epidemiology, 47*(2), 450–459. doi:10.1093/ije/dyx236.

Pounis G, Tabolacci C, Costanzo S, *et al.* (2017). Reduction by coffee consumption of prostate cancer risk: Evidence from the Moli-sani cohort and cellular models. *International Journal of Cancer, 141*(1), 72–82.

Schmit SL, Rennert HS, Rennert G, Gruber SB. (2016). Coffee consumption and the risk of colorectal cancer. *Cancer Epidemiology, Biomarkers & Prevention: A Publication of the American Association for Cancer Research, Cosponsored by the American Society of Preventive Oncology, 25*(4), 634–639. doi:10.1158/1055-9965.EPI-15-0924.

Zamora-Ros R, Luján-Barroso L, Bueno-de-Mesquita HB, *et al.* (2014). Tea and coffee consumption and risk of esophageal cancer: The European prospective investigation into cancer and nutrition study. *International Journal of Cancer, 135*(6), 1470–1479.

Chapter 7

The Sweet Poison: Sugar, a Risk Factor for Cancer Development

As sweet as sugar tastes, the least thing one could expect is the huge health implications. Sugar has become one of the most common household items and its ever presence in food cannot be downplayed. Sugar-containing food provides a unique source of energy for the body cells, which supports human activity and movement. The association of sugar with diabetes is widely known; however, a recent link to cancer development has become the talk of the town. Medical researchers have suspected such link and current studies have provided more insight into this association.

Dr. Tanja Stocks from the University of Umea, Sweden, has conducted a prospective cohort study by following 274,126 men and 275,818 women in Sweden, Austria, and Norway. This research was designed to establish a link between increased blood sugar and cancer risk. The researchers excluded subjects with extreme metabolic parameters and those without smoking data, body mass index (BMI), and glucose levels. As part of the research, the cholesterol, blood pressure, height, and weight of subjects were measured. In the men, 18,621 diagnosed cancer cases were detected with 6,973 cases of fatal cancer death. Also, 11,664 diagnosed cancer cases and 3,098 cases of fatal death were recorded in the women.

Researchers at the University of California, San Francisco, have also confirmed that increased blood sugar is associated with about 35 million deaths globally each year. A strong association between tumor growth and increased blood sugar has been demonstrated by Prof. Don Ayer and colleagues at the Department of Oncological Science, University of Utah. Dr. Thomas Graeber has demonstrated that glucose starvation causes hunger in cancer cells, which leads to the activation of metabolic and signaling mechanisms that ultimately cause the death of cancer cells.

Increased intake of sugar leads to increased blood glucose that nourishes cancer cells to proliferate, differentiate, and metastasize to other distant sites. This mechanism of growth has been attributed to the stimulation of some key metabolic signaling pathways, which lead to the accumulation and activation of growth factors. The growing evidence of association between blood glucose and cancer risk provides a strong platform for extensive cellular and molecular detailing of this mechanism (Fig. 1).

In similar studies, participants who consumed more sugary food and beverages had increased risk of prostate cancer compared with those who consumed less. Specifically, participants who consumed increased amount of fruit juice had 58% increase in prostate cancer risk. Thus, avoiding sugary beverages could be helpful in maintaining good health. A separate study recorded a staggering 23–200% higher cancer risk in participants who consumed sugary beverages in 8 out of 15 studies investigated. There is also evidence demonstrating

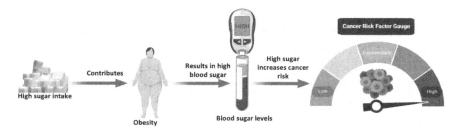

Fig. 1. Increased intake of sugar results in increased cancer risk

that higher sugar intake is associated with fat-associated cancers by 59%. Biliary tract and gall bladder cancer risks were reported to be higher in participants who consumed increased sugar beverages for a particular period of time. In oder to validate the epidemiological findings of the sugar–cancer relationship in meta-analysis studies, a group of researchers investigated if and how glucose affects cancer growth; results were published in the prestigious *Journal of Clinical Investigation.* The authors reported that increased intake of glucose activates tumor-promoting signaling pathways, which results in the production of tumor-promoting proteins involved in driving the growth of cancer cells. Understanding the mechanism of action of these pathways could reveal potential therapeutic targets to help develop effective therapies.

Predominantly, most of the studies described above are epidemiological and hence more mechanistic studies are required to substantiate these important findings. There are several studies that found either weak or no association between cancer risk and juices. Most of the complications are observed with drinks supplemented with artificial sweeteners and sugars. Regardless, there should be regulations on how much sugar could be contained in drinks as well as the type of sugar. This will provide consumers enough information on how much is needed for health benefits and the possible prevention of cancer. Knowledge from such studies could help clinicians plan out a comprehensive care plan taking into consideration the nutrition of cancer patients. Although there is a lot of information about sugary beverages and cancer risk, we have yet to investigate if natural juice from fruits and vegetables either provides good health benefit or compromises the health of consumers. With the emergence of lots of drinks claiming to be organic or natural, studies on natural juice will provide scientific evidence to help regulate their intake.

There is limited evidence to classify sugar as a cancer-causing agent; however, the evidence provided by researchers is enough to support the fact that increased sugar intake is a risk factor for cancer development. Elevated blood sugar level is not a strict determining factor for carcinogenesis since other lifestyle, genetic, and medical conditions play a huge role. It's advisable to minimize the intake of sugar to be on the safer side since cancer development is unpredictable.

Bibliography

Bingham S, Luben R, Welch A, Tasevska N, Wareham N, Khaw KT. (2007). Epidemiologic assessment of sugars consumption using biomarkers: Comparisons of obese and nonobese individuals in the European prospective investigation of cancer Norfolk. *Cancer Epidemiology, Biomarkers & Prevention: A Publication of the American Association for Cancer Research, Cosponsored by the American Society of Preventive Oncology,* *16*(8), 1651–1654. doi:10.1158/1055-9965.EPI-06-1050.

Chazelas E, Srour B, Desmetz E, *et al.* (2019). Sugary drink consumption and risk of cancer: Results from NutriNet-Santé prospective cohort. *BMJ (Clinical Research Ed.), 366,* l2408. doi:10.1136/bmj.l2408.

Fuchs MA, Sato K, Niedzwiecki D, *et al.* (2014). Sugar-sweetened beverage intake and cancer recurrence and survival in CALGB 89803 (Alliance). *PLoS One, 9*(6), e99816. doi:10.1371/journal.pone.0099816

Graham NA, Tahmasian M, Kohli B, *et al.* (2012). Glucose deprivation activates a metabolic and signaling amplification loop leading to cell death. *Molecular Systems Biology, 8,* 589. doi:10.1038/msb.2012.20 https://medicalxpress.com/news/2019-03-evidence-strong-sugar-cancer.html. Retrieved on October 25, 2019.

King MG, Chandran U, Olson SH, *et al.* (2013). Consumption of sugary foods and drinks and risk of endometrial cancer. *Cancer Causes & Control: CCC, 24*(7), 1427–1436. doi:10.1007/s10552-013-0222-0

Larsson SC, Giovannucci EL, Wolk A. (2016). Sweetened beverage consumption and risk of biliary tract and gallbladder cancer in a prospective study. *JNCI: Journal of the National Cancer Institute, 108*(10), djw125. https://doi.org/10.1093/jnci/djw125

Maino Vieytes CA, Taha HM, Burton-Obanla AA, Douglas KG, Arthur AE. (2019). Carbohydrate nutrition and the risk of cancer. *Current Nutrition Reports, 8*(3), 230–239. doi:10.1007/s13668-019-0264-3

Makarem N, Bandera EV, Lin Y, Jacques PF, Hayes RB, Parekh N. (2018). Consumption of sugars, sugary foods and sugary beverages in relation to adiposity-related cancer risk in the Framingham offspring cohort (1991–2013). *Cancer Prevention Research, 11*(6), 347–358. Published online 2018, April 19. doi:10.1158/1940-6207.CAPR-17-0218

Makarem N, Bandera EV, Nicholson JM, Parekh N. (2018). Consumption of sugars, sugary foods, and sugary beverages in relation to cancer risk: A systematic review of longitudinal studies. *Annual Review of Nutrition, 38*(1), 17–39. doi:10.1146/annurev-nutr-082117-051805.

Malik VS, Li Y, Pan A, *et al.* (2019). Long-term consumption of sugar-sweetened and artificially sweetened beverages and risk of mortality in US adults. *Circulation, 139*(18), 2113–2125. doi:10.1161/CIRCULATIONAHA.118.037401.

Miles FL, Neuhouser ML, Zhang ZF. (2018). Concentrated sugars and incidence of prostate cancer in a prospective cohort. *The British Journal of Nutrition, 120*(6), 703–710. doi:10.1017/S0007114518001812.

Navarrete-Muñoz EM, Wark PA, Romaguera D, *et al.* (2016). Sweet-beverage consumption and risk of pancreatic cancer in the European Prospective Investigation into Cancer and Nutrition (EPIC). *The American Journal of Clinical Nutrition, 104*(3), 760–768. doi:10.3945/ajcn.116.130963.

Onodera Y, Nam JM, Bissell MJ. (2014). Increased sugar uptake promotes oncogenesis via EPAC/RAP1 and O-GlcNAc pathways. *The Journal of Clinical Investigation, 124*(1), 367–384. doi:10.1172/JCI63146.

Port AM, Ruth MR, Istfan NW. (2012). Fructose consumption and cancer: Is there a connection? *Current Opinion in Endocrinology, Diabetes, and Obesity, 19*(5), 367–74. doi:10.1097/MED.0b013e328357f0cb.

Prinz P. (2019). The role of dietary sugars in health: Molecular composition or just calories? *European Journal of Clinical Nutrition, 73*(9), 1216–1223. doi:10.1038/s41430-019-0407-z.

Ruxton CH, Gardner EJ, McNulty HM. (2010). Is sugar consumption detrimental to health? A review of the evidence 1995–2006. *Critical Reviews in Food Science and Nutrition, 50*(1), 1–19. doi:10.1080/10408390802248569.

Stocks T, Rapp K, Bjørge T, *et al.* (2009). Blood glucose and risk of incident and fatal cancer in the metabolic syndrome and cancer project (me-can): Analysis of six prospective cohorts. *PLoS Medicine, 6*(12), e1000201. doi:10.1371/journal.pmed.1000201.

University of Utah Health Sciences. (2009). Does sugar feed cancer? *ScienceDaily*. Retrieved on October 25, 2019 from www.sciencedaily.com/releases/2009/08/090817184539.htm.

Wang Z, Uchida K, Ohnaka K, *et al.* (2014). Sugars, sucrose and colorectal cancer risk: The Fukuoka colorectal cancer study. *Scandinavian Journal of Gastroenterology, 49*(5), 581–588. doi:10.3109/00365521.2013.822091.

Chapter 8

Obesity: Pamper Your Weight and Increase Your Cancer Risk by 40%

The acquisition of abnormally high and unhealthy proportion of body fat has been linked to several health complications. This condition is mostly termed as overweight or obesity. Obesity or overweight among US adults aged 20 years or older has increased from 56% between 1988 and 1994 to 68% between 2007 and 2008, according to National Health and Nutrition Examination Survey (NHANES). Many factors contribute to weight gain in people including medical, genetic, emotional, hormonal, environmental, and cultural factors. Researchers normally use the body mass index (BMI) scale to measure obesity; they divide the person's weight (kg) by the height (m) squared. This scale is very reliable to give various categories based on the BMI value: underweight, normal, overweight, and obesity.

Research studies have shown links between obesity and several chronic disorders such as high blood pressure, cardiovascular diseases, and type II diabetes. The increase in recorded obesity cases has prompted scientists to investigate their association with cancer risk. A strong association has been shown between obesity and cancers of the pancreas, breast, esophagus, endometrium, gall bladder, thyroid, colon, rectum, and kidney. A study by Cancer Research UK has shown a 40% higher risk for cancer in obese British women than healthy weight women; 274 out of 1,000 developed a weight-associated cancer in life time.

In a recent study published in the *International Journal of Epidemiology*, the researchers showed that participants who became overweight before 40 years old had an increased risk of developing cancer. From the 220,000 individuals recruited, 27,881 of them were diagnosed of cancer, of which 35% were obesity-related. This provides a strong association between obesity and cancer risk. In 2007, the National Cancer Institute (NCI) Surveillance, Epidemiology, and End Results (SEER) estimated that 34,000 newly diagnosed cancer cases in American men and 50,500 cases diagnosed in women were associated with obesity. This data further projected additional 500,000 cases by 2030 if the existing trends continue. In 2014, overweight and obesity were associated with 13 types of cancer in the United States, which represent 40% of all cancers diagnosed. These include endometrial, ovarian, breast, liver, kidney, colorectal, pancreatic, gall bladder, thyroid, esophageal, and gastric cancers (Fig. 1).

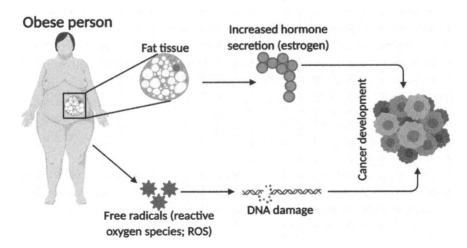

Fig. 1.   Obesity has the ability to increase cancer risk by 40%

Obesity leads to increased production of inflammatory and growth factors that drive tumor-promoting signaling. This can result in the development of cancer at many sites in the body. Understanding the crosstalk between these signals could lead to interventional therapies that could be exploited to enhance patient survival. Other studies have shown that obesity is associated with the less aggressive form of ovarian cancer called non-high grade serous ovarian carcinoma. Although less aggressive, there are not many treatment options since most of the research attention is focused on the more aggressive type. In addition to ovarian cancer, obesity has been associated with increased risk of subtype-specific breast cancer especially estrogen positive (ER+) and negative (ER−) breast cancer.

Obesity is not a proof of cancer, but rather increases cancer risk through some suggested mechanisms. Fat tissues/cells produce excess estrogen and leptin that are associated with increased risk of developing breast and endometrial cancers. These hormones are released into the blood stream and travel to most parts of the body, hence exposing the victim to different types of cancer. Chronic low level inflammation in obese patients could also trigger the development of tumor. Fat cells have both direct and indirect effects on tumor growth factors as well as regulators that may promote the development of certain cancers. Oxidative stress, which is high in obese victims, generates free radicals that cause detrimental effects to cells. This can cause mutations and then increase the risk of tumor growth.

Pampering your weight comes with serious complications hence the need to avoid that habit. Your ability to avoid being overweight could help decrease your cancer risk. Developing the attitude of eating considerable amount of vegetables, fruits, lean protein, and whole grains could help maintain a healthy weight. Decreasing the level of high-calorie containing diets and drinks with increased levels of physical activity could be a very good weight management plan. Regardless, this could also be influenced by sex, genes, race, and other medical treatments. Obesity is not the only contributing factor to developing cancer; however, your ability to maintain a healthy weight provides some level of protection against cancer.

Bibliography

Bjørge T, Häggström C, Ghaderi S, *et al.* (2019). BMI and weight changes and risk of obesity-related cancers: A pooled European cohort study. *International Journal of Epidemiology, 48*(6), 1872–1885. doi:10.1093/ije/dyz188.

Calle EE, Rodriguez C, Walker-Thurmond K, Thun MJ. (2003). Overweight, obesity, and mortality from cancer in a prospectively studied cohort of U.S. adults. *New England Journal of Medicine, 348*(17), 1625–1638.

Campbell PT, Jacobs ET, Ulrich CM, *et al.* (2010). Case-control study of overweight, obesity, and colorectal cancer risk, overall and by tumor microsatellite instability status. *Journal of the National Cancer Institute, 102*(6), 391–400. doi:10.1093/jnci/djq011.

Chen Y, Liu L, Wang X, *et al.* (2013). Body mass index and risk of gastric cancer: A meta-analysis of a population with more than ten million from 24 prospective studies. *Cancer Epidemiology, Biomarkers & Prevention, 22*(8), 1395–1408.

Chen Y, Wang X, Wang J, Yan Z, Luo J. (2012). Excess body weight and the risk of primary liver cancer: An updated meta-analysis of prospective studies. *European Journal of Cancer, 48*(14), 2137–2145.

Collaborative Group on Epidemiological Studies of Ovarian Cancer. (2012). Ovarian cancer and body size: Individual participant meta-analysis including 25,157 women with ovarian cancer from 47 epidemiological studies. *PLoS Medicine, 9*(4), e1001200. doi:10.1371/journal.pmed.1001200.

Cox-Martin E, Trahan LH, Cox MG, Dougherty PM, Lai EA, Novy DM. (2017). Disease burden and pain in obese cancer patients with chemo-therapy-induced peripheral neuropathy. *Supportive Care in Cancer: Official Journal of the Multinational Association of Supportive Care in Cancer, 25*(6), 1873–1879. doi:10.1007/s00520-017-3571-5.

Dixon SC, Nagle CM, Thrift AP, *et al.* (2016). Adult body mass index and risk of ovarian cancer by subtype: A Mendelian randomization study. *International Journal of Epidemiology, 45*(3), 884–895. doi:10.1093/ije/dyw158.

Gacci M, Sebastianelli A, Salvi M, *et al.* (2014). Role of abdominal obesity for functional outcomes and complications in men treated with radical prostatectomy for prostate cancer: Results of the Multicenter Italian

Report on Radical Prostatectomy (MIRROR) study. *Scandinavian Journal of Urology, 48*(2), 138–145.

Gregor MF, Hotamisligil GS. (2011). Inflammatory mechanisms in obesity. *Annual Review of Immunology, 29*, 415–445.

Himbert C, Delphan M, Scherer D, Bowers LW, Hursting S, Ulrich CM. (2017). Signals from the adipose microenvironment and the obesity-cancer link — A systematic review. *Cancer Prevention Research (Philadelphia, PA.), 10*(9), 494–506. doi:10.1158/1940-6207.CAPR-16-0322.

https://www.cancer.gov/about-cancer/causes-prevention/risk/obesity/obesity-fact-sheet. Retrieved on October 28, 2019.

https://www.cancerresearchuk.org/about-cancer/causes-of-cancer/obesity-weight-and-cancer. Retrieved on October 28, 2019.

https://www.cdc.gov/media/releases/2017/p1003-vs-cancer-obesity.html. Retrieved on October 28, 2019.

https://www.cdc.gov/nchs/data/factsheets/factsheet_nhanes.htm. Retrieved on October 28, 2019.

Kerlikowske K, Gard CC, Tice JA, *et al.* (2016). Risk factors that increase risk of estrogen receptor-positive and -negative breast cancer. *Journal of the National Cancer Institute, 109*(5), djw276. doi:10.1093/jnci/djw276.

Lashinger LM, Ford NA, Hursting SD. (2014). Interacting inflammatory and growth factor signals underlie the obesity-cancer link. *The Journal of Nutrition, 144*(2), 109–113. doi:10.3945/jn.113.178533.

Li L, Gan Y, Li W, Wu C, Lu Z. (2016). Overweight, obesity and the risk of gallbladder and extrahepatic bile duct cancers: A meta-analysis of observational studies. *Obesity (Silver Spring), 24*(8), 1786–1802.

Ma Y, Yang Y, Wang F, *et al.* (2013). Obesity and risk of colorectal cancer: A systematic review of prospective studies. *PLoS One, 8*(1), e53916.

Nagle CM, Dixon SC, Jensen A, *et al.* (2015). Obesity and survival among women with ovarian cancer: Results from the Ovarian Cancer Association Consortium. *British Journal of Cancer, 113*(5), 817–826. doi:10.1038/bjc.2015.245.

Roberts DL, Dive C, Renehan AG. (2010). Biological mechanisms linking obesity and cancer risk: New perspectives. *Annual Review of Medicine, 61*, 301–316.

Seo BR, Bhardwaj P, Choi S. (2015). Obesity-dependent changes in interstitial ECM mechanics promote breast tumorigenesis. *Science Translational Medicine, 7*(301), 301ra130.

Shu X, Wu L, Khankari NK, *et al.* (2019). Associations of obesity and circulating insulin and glucose with breast cancer risk: A Mendelian randomization analysis. *International Journal of Epidemiology, 48*(3), 795–806.

Strong AL, Burow ME, Gimble JM, Bunnell BA. (2015). Concise review: The obesity cancer paradigm: Exploration of the interactions and cross-talk with adipose stem cells. *Stem Cells (Dayton, Ohio), 33*(2), 318–326. doi:10.1002/stem.1857.

Chapter 9

Super Foods that Offer Anticancer Benefits

Cancer treatment is very expensive and could cost $90,000 just to increase survival by 14 months. Such an amount is ridiculously high and could only be afforded by some few groups of people. This might be a contributing factor why cancer is still on the surge despite relentless effort to discover novel therapeutic options. Cost-effective cancer preventive measures could be located in your fridges. The vegetables and fruits in the fridge could provide some level of protection against the growth of cancer and other chronic diseases. More research scientists have now directed their studies toward developing cost-effective treatment modalities through the exploration of some vegetables and fruits. Most of these fruits and vegetables also help in the management of pain associated with cancer treatment.

Ginger

Ginger extracts have been proven to be of therapeutic importance against cancer. Researchers from King Abdul-Aziz University, Saudi Arabia, have explored the anticancer properties of ginger extracts and have also confirmed their superiority over any drug currently in the market for breast cancer treatment. Extracts from ginger have also shown great therapeutic promise in a plethora of gastrointestinal cancers and ovarian cancer as well as other inflammatory disorders. In a mouse study at the Hormel Institute, University of Minnesota, gingerol, a phytonutrient, has been shown to be very effective against colorectal cancer treatment. A similar anticancer property of gingerol was demonstrated by Dr. Rebecca Lui at the University of Michigan where gingerol induced programmed cell death (apoptosis) and self-digestion (autophagocytosis) in ovarian cancer cells. In a comprehensive review, it was shown that gingerol, an extract of ginger, acts by modulating both proliferative and anti-tumor signaling pathways. A 56% reduction in mice prostate cancer was shown in a study conducted at the Georgia State University where whole ginger extracts were used as treatments. Most importantly, the ginger extracts did not exert any toxicity on the normal cells (Fig. 1).

Ginger produces bioactive antioxidants (6-gingerol and 6-shogaol) that are potentially packaged and transported via nano-particles that have been shown to reduce inflammation in the colon, a response that has the potential of reducing cancer development. These nanoparticles showed no toxicity on normal cells but exerted therapeutic effects against colitis and inflammation-induced cancers. This presents as a novel therapeutic strategy to maximize treatment efficiency while preventing adverse side effects. Dietary ginger activates programmed cell death pathways that contribute to the killing of the aggressive form of breast cancer (triple negative

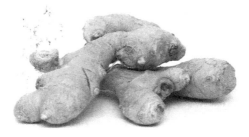

Fig. 1.   Ginger

breast cancer) cells and non-small cell lung cancer cells. Extracts from ginger such as gingerol have been shown to lower the levels of tumor-promoting enzymes (cyclooxygenase; COX-1) in colorectal cancers.

In a mice study, 6-shogaol, an active constituent of dietary ginger, provided significant anticancer effects on cancer development as well as prevented lung metastasis. This is done through the inhibition of inflammatory chemicals called CC-chemokine ligand 2 (CCL2). Using experimental rats, zingerone (an active component of ginger) demonstrated chemopreventive properties against mammary cancer cells via programmed cell death (apoptosis). So far, extracts from dietary ginger have demonstrated no side effects to normal tissues while exerting significant cancer prevention properties. These effects have been shown in a plethora of cancers such as breast, ovarian, lung, colorectal, esophageal, prostate, and pancreatic cancers. It is yet to be investigated if ginger extracts could be used in the clinics or administered together with other cancer therapeutic drugs. With this strong correlative evidence, addition of ginger in moderation to our meals could be very beneficial to our health.

Cruciferous Vegetables — Broccoli

Scientists have explored cruciferous vegetables like broccoli to identify some phytonutrients — indoles and sulforaphane — that could be used for cancer treatment. Emily Ho of Linus Pauling Institute, Oregon State University, has revealed the anticancer properties of sulforaphane against prostate cancer. Sulforaphane has the ability to induce phase-2-enzymes in the liver that help fight carcinogens and also inhibit histone deacetylase (HDAC) enzymes, which ultimately restores cells to normal function. Its capacity to induce selective killing makes it an attractive and promising therapeutic agent. A mouse study conducted at the University of Michigan Comprehensive Cancer Center has also demonstrated the efficacy of sulforaphane against cancer stem cells (a small population of stubborn cells that fuel cancer growth). This is very promising since most chemotherapeutic

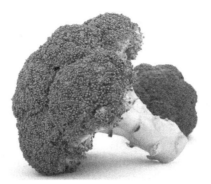

Fig. 2. Broccoli

agents are unable to kill these cancer stem cells. Most studies have shown broccoli to be useful in the treatment of breast, prostate, liver, lung, bladder, and stomach cancers. In a study published in the journal *Science*, extracts from broccoli reactivated a tumor suppressor gene called *PTEN*, which then mitigated the cancer development (Fig. 2).

Isothiocyanates derived from cruciferous vegetables such as broccoli promote tumor killing signals that result in the inhibition of bladder cancer using cell lines and animal models. In a clinical trial registered at clinicaltrials.gov as NCT01950143, it is reported that consuming glucoraphanin-rich broccoli soup regulated gene expression in the prostate of men, resulting in reduced cancer progression. Apart from the genetic regulation properties of cruciferous vegetables, researchers have also reported epigenetic regulation by extracts from these vegetables. Extracts from cruciferous vegetables epigenetically regulate genes involved in tumor development. Such changes result in the suppression of tumor-promoting genes especially in breast cancer.

Cruciferous vegetables therefore present as an inexpensive means of suppressing cancer growth. It will also be beneficial if cruciferous vegetables such as broccoli are genetically edited to produce more of the bioactive components such as glucoraphanin, which could be exploited for their health benefits. With such significant evidence, there is no doubt meals containing broccoli could be beneficial to our health.

Tomatoes

Tomatoes are the second most widely eaten vegetables in the United States and contain a pigment called lycopene that contributes to the red color of vegetables and fruits (Fig. 3). Lycopene has been identified as an antioxidant that neutralizes the effects of free radicals. The American Institute for Cancer Research (AICR) has named tomatoes as one of the superfoods that contain anticancer properties. Lycopene induces self-destruction procedures (apoptosis) in cancer cells especially in prostate cancer where a reduction in cancer risk has been shown. In a review by Edward Giovannucci from the University of Harvard, he showed data examining the therapeutic effects of lycopene on prostate cancer. Researchers in the United Kingdom have revealed a 20% reduction in prostate cancer risk but however, recommended balancing a healthy diet with active lifestyle. Lycopene has also been implicated in the treatment of lung, endometrial, stomach, and prostate cancers. Although tomatoes have significant health benefits, iron-containing foods such as cereals cancel out the benefits of lycopene and thus minimize the anticancer properties of tomatoes.

In a mouse study, lycopene extracted from dietary tomato reduced the aggressiveness of prostate cancer as well as improved the overall survival of animals implanted with prostate cancer. Carotenoid- and polyphenol-rich tomatoes inhibit tumor-promoting signals, leading to a reduced risk of chronic diseases and liver cancers. In a separate animal study, dietary tomato powder

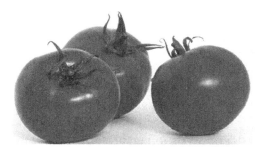

Fig. 3.   Tomatoes

suppressed liver cancer induced by high fat diet. This happened via alteration in the gut microbiota (bacteria composition in the intestines). The cancer protection properties of dietary tomatoes have been implicated in other cancers such as ovarian, endometroid, colorectal, brain, and breast cancers. Impressively, the bioactive constituents in the dietary tomatoes have no toxicity against normal tissues, thus, presenting as a novel therapeutic agent for cancer treatment.

Although these findings are promising, understanding the mechanisms of action of the various bioactive constituents is key to developing effective therapeutic strategies. Scientists could genetically modify tomatoes to produce more of the bioactive agents involved in offering cancer protection. This could contribute to the availability of treatments at a lower price, which could be afforded by all patients regardless of economic status. Establishing a medically recommended dosage of dietary tomatoes will be essential to both clinicians and patients in improving the survival of patients. Further clinical studies are needed to examine the efficacy of dietary tomatoes alone or its combination with other treatments such as immunotherapy, chemotherapy, radiotherapy, surgery, or hormonal treatments.

Moderate consumption of tomatoes in households is therefore recommended and families could plant this wonderful fruit/vegetable in their backyard gardens. Regardless, consumers should not substitute tomatoes with their prescribed medication. Patients could seek advice from their clinicians as to whether they can combine tomatoes-rich diets with their prescribed medications.

Berries

Gary D. Stoner, PhD, Medical College of Wisconsin, led a study which revealed that berries contain increased amount of anthocyanins and ellagitannins that are effective against tumor growth and angiogenesis (developing new vessels to feed tumor cells). These phytonutrients are reported to decrease esophageal cancer growth by 30–70% in rats, 80% reduction in colon cancer, and 36% reduction in rectal

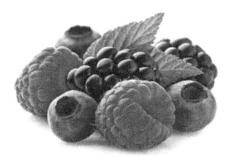

Fig. 4. Berries

polyps. Harini Aiyer, PhD, Postdoctoral Research Fellow, Lombardi Cancer Center, George Town University of Medicine, has also shown 60–70% decrease in ER+ breast tumor volumes. Extracts from blueberries have also been shown to sensitize cervical cancer cells to radiation therapy, thus, serving as a potential agent to increase the overall survival of cervical cancer patients (Fig. 4).

Bioactive constituents of berries provide both therapeutic and preventive effects against colon cancer by suppressing inflammation, tumor growth, and metastasis (spread to other sites). There are findings to also support the inhibition of angiogenesis by edible berries. Using mice and cells, researchers have also demonstrated significant findings where breast cancer growth, metastasis, and aggressiveness were halted by strawberries. This molecular and cellular evidence has been translated into humans where few clinical trials have shown significant promise in the therapeutic and preventive effects of berries.

Understanding how berries exert their therapeutic effects is critical to developing potent cancer treatments. As to whether berries could be administered as a single treatment or combined with other FDA-approved drugs is yet to be investigated. Regulating the dosage of the active components in berries will maximize therapeutic successes and minimize adverse side effects. Depending on the type of berry, there are varying amount and potencies of their bioactive compounds against cancer. Thus, the efficacy of protection you gain depends on the type of berries eaten. Lots of studies are therefore needed in this area of research to demonstrate the levels of protection provided by each type of berry to guide consumers on which ones to be bought and eaten. This will also provide valuable information to biopharmaceutical industries and clinicians on how to manage patients taking into consideration their nutritional benefits and drug combinations. These promising results make berries potential anticancer fruits that should be often seen in fridges across homes.

Allium Vegetables — Garlic

As indicated by the Iowa Women's Health Study, increased intake of garlic cuts down colon cancer risk by 50%. The mechanism of action has been attributed to anticancer effects of some phytochemicals like quercetin, allixin, allicin, alliin, and allyl identified in garlic. In a population-based case study in Chinese population, Zi-Yi Jin reported an association between increased garlic intake and 44% reduction in lung cancer risk. Moreover, 30% reduction was also identified in smokers. Other studies have shown similar therapeutic promises in esophageal, colon, breast, and stomach cancers. Garlic contains phytonutrients that help DNA repair, boost enzymes that deactivate carcinogens as well as inhibit enzymes that activate cancer-causing genes. Garlic extracts also minimize the ability for cancer cells to stimulate new blood vessels, a phenomenon that is used by cancer cells to spread. Also, garlic offers health benefits against other inflammatory and chronic disorders (Fig. 5).

Dietary bioactive diallyl trisulfide (BDT) from *Allium* vegetables such as garlic and onions regulates many cancer pathways involved in apoptosis, invasion, angiogenesis, metastasis, and cell cycle that ultimately contribute to reduction in cancer risk and development. In animal studies, other bioactive agents from garlic exerted significant antimetastatic effects against prostate cancer. Selenium-rich onions and garlic have also shown therapeutic promise in different types of cancers. Garlic has more selenium compared with onions and as such exerts more therapeutic effects. Although selenium toxicity in tissues is a huge concern, dietary selenium from garlic

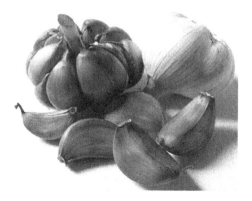

Fig. 5. Garlic

showed no organ accumulation, making it a reliable therapeutic candidate. Beside anticancer properties, bioactive components from garlic have the ability to regulate immune functions such as T lymphocytes and natural killer (NK) cells. Enhancing the functions of these cells provides efficient immune surveillance in the tumor microenvironment, helping in the elimination of tumor cells. Such antitumor effects have been demonstrated against stomach and colorectal cancers.

A few of these epidemiological and preclinical studies have been translated into the clinics for trials. Increased garlic consumption of 20 g/day reduced the risk of gastric and colorectal cancers (digestive cancers) compared with the control cohorts who took less or nothing. Regardless of the therapeutic promises of garlic and other *Allium* vegetables, there are still discrepancies in the research findings. Most of the studies do not clearly state whether the garlic used is cooked or raw. This piece of information could be helpful to consumers in order to achieve the full benefits of these vegetables. Also, other confounding factors such as sex, dose differences, race, and mode of cooking should be addressed to substantiate the potency of dietary garlic in the prevention and protection against cancer.

The above scientific evidence is a testimony why garlic should be made part of our daily meal. In the case of cancer patients, permission should be sought from healthcare providers before combining increased garlic consumption with prescribed medication to avoid contraindications.

Beans

Beans come in various shapes, sizes, and colors (Fig. 6). In addition to the fact that beans are a rich source of protein, studies have revealed they also contain anticancer properties. Beans are rich in folate and dietary fiber that help to improve healthy DNA, control weight gain, and decrease the risk of colorectal cancer. Researchers at the University College London have identified inositol pentakisphosphate in beans that reduces tumor growth. This active compound inhibits oncogenic enzymes that ultimately halt cancer growth. The phytonutrient sensitizes ovarian and lung cancer cells to chemotherapeutic agents. A 42% reduction in colon cancer risk has also been reported in a study conducted at the Loma Linda University.

Most of the phytochemicals identified are antioxidants and they neutralize the damaging effects of free radicals. This prevents DNA damages that could result in cancer. Dr. James Watson, the codiscoverer of the DNA structure, has urged scientists to reconsider the role of antioxidants else the cure for many cancers will remain elusive. According to Dr. James Watson, antioxidants might also have a role

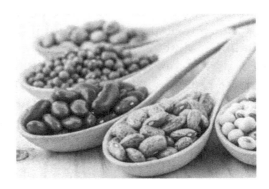

Fig. 6. Beans

to play in cancer development as free radicals are needed to cause destruction of tumor cells or apoptosis of dysfunctional cells that pose threat to survival.

Higher intake of dry beans has been shown to be associated with a reduction in advanced colorectal recurrence. In a randomized controlled trial, 35 g/day of beans showed significant chemopreventive properties against colorectal cancers. As to whether antioxidants contribute to cancer development, substantial information is needed to confirm that. However, numerous studies have confirmed the anticancer properties of antioxidants. Regardless, more molecular and cellular details are needed to provide convincing mechanisms of action of these phytonutrients. Fruits and veggies should remain important components of our daily meals as they provide incredible health benefits including anticancer properties.

Ginseng

Ginseng is the root of *Panax* plants with three main characterized types: Chinese ginseng (*P. notoginseng*), Korean ginseng (*P. ginseng*), and American ginseng (*P. quinquefolius*). Ginseng is highly enriched with bioactive components such as ginsenosides and gintonin that have shown significant health benefits for centuries. This is mostly patronized in Asia especially China and Korea where it has been shown to be effective in the treatment of heart diseases, erectile dysfunction, fatigue, viral infections, and high blood pressures. Regardless of its potential health benefits, ginseng has not been approved by FDA and could only be classified as a dietary supplement (Fig. 7).

Recently, there has been lots of literature reporting about the cancer preventive and protective properties of ginseng. Ginseng is implicated in reducing inflammation, oxidative stress, metastasis, angiogenesis, and proliferation resulting in suppression of tumor growth as well as cancer risk. Polysaccharide (PGP2a) extracted from the root of *Panax ginseng* induces programmed cell death of human gastric cancer cells. PGP2a improves immune function by activating NK cells, tumor killing macrophages, T cells as well as

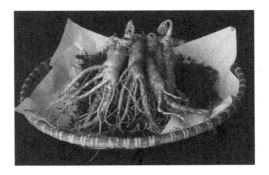

Fig. 7. Ginseng

inducing tumor killing chemicals — responses that contribute immensely to tumor killing and suppression of metastasis. Ginsenoside, another bioactive agent in ginseng, demonstrates chemoprevention properties against ovarian cancer and the aggressive form of breast cancer (triple negative) as well as significantly suppresses metastasis in colorectal cancer.

In a mice experiment, administering ginseng orally reduced inflammation and improved the gut microbiota composition, which suppressed inflammation-induced colon cancer. In a multisite double-blind randomized trial, 2,000 mg daily of ginseng over an eight-week period improved cancer-related fatigue (CRF). This is suggestive that ginseng not only protects against cancer development but also has the ability to suppress fatigues caused by cancer. Although these findings are exciting and promising, there is the urgent need to investigate the quality, safety, and efficacy of the various types of ginseng. This will provide a recommended dose that could be used worldwide to achieve similar therapeutic effects. Ginseng shows no toxicity against normal tissues hence presents as a reliable therapeutic agent. Further studies are needed to test if ginseng bioactive agents could be used individually or in combination with other FDA-approved drugs or conventional treatments such as surgery, chemotherapy, or radiotherapy.

It's incredible how the everyday foods in our fridges could be life saving. Care should be taken not to abuse their intake since too much of anything has severe consequences. Seeking advice

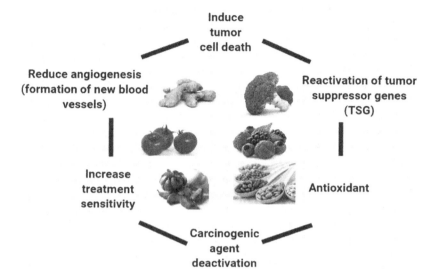

Fig. 8. These foods provide chemopreventive advantages through a plethora of mechanisms

from nutritional experts can go a long way to helping achieve the full benefits of these power foods (Fig. 8).

Bibliography

Abbaoui B, Lucas CR, Riedl KM, Clinton SK, Mortazavi A. (2018). Cruciferous vegetables, isothiocyanates, and bladder cancer prevention. *Molecular Nutrition & Food Research*, *62*(18), e1800079. doi:10.1002/mnfr.201800079.

Abbas A, Hall JA, Patterson WL 3rd, *et al.* (2016). Sulforaphane modulates telomerase activity via epigenetic regulation in prostate cancer cell lines. *Biochemistry and Cell Biology*, *94*, 71–81.

Afrin S, Giampieri F, Gasparrini M, *et al.* (2016). Chemopreventive and therapeutic effects of edible berries: A focus on colon cancer prevention and treatment. *Molecules*, *21*(2), 169. doi:10.3390/molecules21020169.

Aiyer HS, Kichambare S, Gupta RC. (2008). Prevention of oxidative DNA damage by bioactive berry components. *Nutrition and Cancer*, *60*(Suppl. 1), 36–42. doi:10.1080/01635580802398448.

Aiyer HS, Warri AM, Woode DR, Hilakivi-Clarke L, Clarke R. (2012). Influence of berry polyphenols on receptor signaling and cell-death pathways: Implications for breast cancer prevention. *Journal of Agricultural and Food Chemistry, 60*(23), 5693–5708. doi:10.1021/jf204084f.

Baby B, Antony P, Vijayan R. (2018). Antioxidant and anticancer properties of berries. *Critical Reviews in Food Science and Nutrition, 58*(15), 2491–2507. doi:10.1080/10408398.2017.1329198.

Baliga MS, Haniadka R, Pereira MM, *et al.* (2011). Update on the chemopreventive effects of ginger and its phytochemicals. *Critical Reviews in Food Science and Nutrition, 51*(6), 499–523. doi:10.1080/10408391003698669.

Barton DL, Liu H, Dakhil SR, *et al.* (2013). Wisconsin Ginseng (*Panax quinquefolius*) to improve cancer-related fatigue: A randomized, double-blind trial, N07C2. *Journal of the National Cancer Institute, 105*(16), 1230–1238. doi:10.1093/jnci/djt181.

Borresen EC, Brown DG, Harbison G, *et al.* (2016). A randomized controlled trial to increase navy bean or rice bran consumption in colorectal cancer survivors. *Nutrition and Cancer, 68*(8), 1269–1280. doi:10.1080/01635581.2016.1224370.

Borresen EC, Gundlach KA, Wdowik M, Rao S, Brown RJ, Ryan EP. (2014). Feasibility of increased navy bean powder consumption for primary and secondary colorectal cancer prevention. *Current Nutrition and Food Science, 10*(2), 112–119. doi:10.2174/1573401310666140306005934.

Chen L, Xin X, Yuan Q, Su D, Liu W. (2014, January 30). Phytochemical properties and antioxidant capacities of various colored berries. *Journal of the Science of Food and Agriculture, 94*(2), 180–188.

Clarke JD, Dashwood RH, Ho E. (2008). Multi-targeted prevention of cancer by sulforaphane. *Cancer Letters, 269*(2), 291–304. doi:10.1016/j.canlet.2008.04.018.

Clement IP, Donald J. (1994). Lisk, enrichment of selenium in allium vegetables for cancer prevention. *Carcinogenesis, 15*(9), 1881–1885. doi:10.1093/carcin/15.9.1881.

Davidson KT, Zhu Z, Bai Q, Xiao H, Wakefield MR, Fang Y. (2019). Blueberry as a potential radiosensitizer for treating cervical cancer. *Pathology & Oncology Research, 25*, 81–88. doi:10.1007/s12253-017-0319-y.

de Lima RMT, Dos Reis AC, de Menezes APM, *et al.* (2018, July 16). Protective and therapeutic potential of ginger (*Zingiber officinale*) extract and [6]-gingerol in cancer: A comprehensive review. *Phytotherapy Research. 32*(10), 1885–1907. doi:10.1002/ptr.6134.

Elkady AI, Abuzinadah OA, Baeshen NA, Rahmy TR. (2012). Differential control of growth, apoptotic activity, and gene expression in human breast cancer cells by extracts derived from medicinal herbs *Zingiber officinale. Journal of Biomedicine & Biotechnology, 2012,* 614356. doi:10.1155/2012/614356.

Fleischauer AT, Poole C, Arab, L. (2000). Garlic consumption and cancer prevention: Meta-analyses of colorectal and stomach cancers. *The American Journal of Clinical Nutrition, 72*(4), 1047–1052. doi:10.1093/ajcn/72.4.1047.

Fu J, Chen H, Soroka DN, Warin RF, Sang S. (2014). Cysteine-conjugated metabolites of ginger components, shogaols, induce apoptosis through oxidative stress-mediated p53 pathway in human colon cancer cells. *Journal of Agricultural and Food Chemistry, 62*(20), 4632–4642. doi:10.1021/jf501351r.

Gan H, Zhang Y, Zhou Q, *et al.* (2019). Zingerone induced caspase-dependent apoptosis in MCF-7 cells and prevents 7,12-dimethylbenz(a)anthracene induced mammary carcinogenesis in experimental rats. *Journal of Biochemical and Molecular Toxicology, 33,* e22387. doi:10.1002/jbt.22387.

Giovannucci E, Rimm EB, Liu Y, Stampfer MJ, Willett WC. (2002). A prospective study of tomato products, lycopene, and prostate cancer risk. *Journal of the National Cancer Institute, 94*(5), 391–398.

Graff RE, Pettersson A, Lis RT, *et al.* (2016). Dietary lycopene intake and risk of prostate cancer defined by ERG protein expression. *The American Journal of Clinical Nutrition, 103*(3), 851–860. doi:10.3945/ajcn.115.118703.

Herr I, Büchler MW. (2010). Dietary constituents of broccoli and other cruciferous vegetables: Implications for prevention and therapy of cancer. *Cancer Treatment Reviews, 36*(5), 377–383.

Holzapfel NP, Holzapfel BM, Theodoropoulos C, *et al.* (2016). Lycopene's effects on cancer cell functions within monolayer and spheroid cultures. *Nutrition and Cancer, 68*(2), 350–363. doi:10.1080/01635581.2016.1150498.

Hong Y, Fan D. (2019). Ginsenoside Rk1 induces cell cycle arrest and apoptosis in MDA-MB-231 triple negative breast cancer cells. *Toxicology.* doi:10.1016/j.tox.2019.02.010.

Howard EW, Ling MT, Chua CW, Cheung HW, Wang X, Wong YC. (2007). Garlic-derived S-allylmercaptocysteine is a novel in vivo antimetastatic agent for androgen-independent prostate cancer. *Clinical Cancer Research: An Official Journal of the American Association for Cancer Research, 13*(6), 1847–1856. doi:10.1158/1078-0432.CCR-06-2074.

Hsu A, Wong CP, Yu Z, Williams DE, Dashwood RH, Ho E. (2011). Promoter de-methylation of cyclin D2 by sulforaphane in prostate cancer cells. *Clinical Epigenetics, 3*(1), 3. doi:10.1186/1868-7083-3-3.

Hsu YL, Hung J-Y, Tsai Y-M, *et al.* (2015). 6-Shogaol, an active constituent of dietary ginger, impairs cancer development and lung metastasis by inhibiting the secretion of CC-chemokine ligand 2 (CCL2) in tumor-associated dendritic cells. *Journal of Agricultural and Food Chemistry, 63*(6), 1730–1738. doi:10.1021/jf504934m.

https://www.aicr.org/foods-that-fight-cancer/garlic.html. Retrieved on 2019, October 28.

https://www.aicr.org/foods-that-fight-cancer/legumes.html. Retrieved on 2019, October 28.

https://www.aicr.org/foods-that-fight-cancer/tomatoes.html. Retrieved on 2019, October 28.

https://www.aicr.org/publications/newsletter/2013-spring-119/berries-seem-to-burst-with-cancer-prevention.html. Retrieved on October 28, 2019.

https://www.bbc.com/news/health-28950093. Retrieved on October 28, 2019 .

James D, Devaraj S, Bellur P, Lakkanna S, Vicini J, Boddupalli S. (2012). Novel concepts of broccoli sulforaphanes and disease: Induction of phase II antioxidant and detoxification enzymes by enhanced-glucoraphanin broccoli. *Nutrition Reviews, 70*(11), 654–665.

Jiang Y, Turgeon DK, Wright BD, *et al.* (2013). Effect of ginger root on cyclooxygenase-1 and 15-hydroxyprostaglandin dehydrogenase expression in colonic mucosa of humans at normal and increased risk for colorectal cancer. *European Journal of Cancer Prevention: The Official Journal of the European Cancer Prevention Organisation (ECP), 22*(5), 455–460. doi:10.1097/CEJ.0b013e32835c829b.

Jin ZY, Wu M, Han RQ, *et al.* (2013). Raw garlic consumption as a protective factor for lung cancer, a population-based case-control study in a Chinese population. *Cancer Prevention Research (Philadelphia, PA.), 6*(7), 711–718. doi:10.1158/1940-6207.CAPR-13-0015.

Karna P, Chagani S, Gundala SR, *et al.* (2012). Benefits of whole ginger extract in prostate cancer. *The British Journal of Nutrition, 107*(4), 473–484. doi:10.1017/S0007114511003308.

Kristo AS, Klimis-Zacas D, Sikalidis AK. (2016). Protective role of dietary berries in cancer. *Antioxidants (Basel, Switzerland), 5*(4), 37. doi:10.3390/antiox5040037.

Kweon SS, Shu XO, Xiang Y, *et al.* (2013). Intake of specific nonfermented soy foods may be inversely associated with risk of distal gastric cancer in a Chinese population. *The Journal of Nutrition, 143*(11), 1736–1742. doi:10.3945/jn.113.177675.

Lanza E, Hartman TJ, Albert PS, *et al.* (2006). High dry bean intake and reduced risk of advanced colorectal adenoma recurrence among participants in the polyp prevention trial. *The Journal of Nutrition, 136*(7), 1896–1903. doi:10.1093/jn/136.7.1896.

Lee YR, Chen M, Lee JD, *et al.* (2019). Reactivation of PTEN tumor suppressor for cancer treatment through inhibition of a MYC-WWP1 inhibitory pathway. *Science, 364*(6441), pii: eaau0159. doi:10.1126/science.aau0159.

Li C, Tian Z-N, Cai J-P, *et al.* (2014). *Panax ginseng* polysaccharide induces apoptosis by targeting Twist/AKR1C2/NF-1 pathway in human gastric cancer. *Carbohydrate Polymers, 102*, 103–109.

Li Y, Zhang T, Korkaya H, *et al.* (2010). Sulforaphane, a dietary component of broccoli/broccoli sprouts, inhibits breast cancer stem cells. *Clinical Cancer Research, 16*(9), 2580. doi:10.1158/1078-0432.CCR-09-2937.

Li Y, Buckhaults P, Li S, Tollefsbol T. (2018). Temporal efficacy of a sulforaphane-based broccoli sprout diet in prevention of breast cancer through modulation of epigenetic mechanisms. *Cancer Prevention Research, 11*(8), 451–464. doi:10.1158/1940-6207.CAPR-17-0423.

Majeed F, Malik FZ, Ahmed Z, Afreen A, Afzal MN, Khalid N. (2018). Ginseng phytochemicals as therapeutics in oncology: Recent perspectives. *Biomedicine & Pharmacotherapy, 100*, 52–63. doi:10.1016/j.biopha.2018.01.155.

Martí R, Roselló S, Cebolla-Cornejo J. (2016). Tomato as a source of carotenoids and polyphenols targeted to cancer prevention. *Cancers, 8*(6), 58. doi:10.3390/cancers8060058.

McCullough ML, Jacobs EJ, Shah R, Campbell PT, Gapstur SM. (2012). Garlic consumption and colorectal cancer risk in the CPS-II Nutrition Cohort. *Cancer Causes and Control, 23*(10), 1643–1651.

Miraghajani M, Rafie N, Hajianfar H, Larijani B, Azadbakht L. (2018). Aged garlic and cancer: A systematic review. *International Journal of Preventive Medicine, 9*, 84. doi:10.4103/ijpvm.IJPVM_437_17.

Murthy HN, Dandin VS, Park SY, Paek KY. (2018). Quality, safety and efficacy profiling of ginseng adventitious roots produced *in vitro. Applied Microbiology and Biotechnology.*

Nedungadi D, Binoy A, Vinod V, *et al.* (2019). Ginger extract activates caspase independent paraptosis in cancer cells via ER stress, mitochondrial dysfunction, AIF translocation and DNA damage. *Nutrition and Cancer.* doi:10.1080/01635581.2019.1685113.

Oh J, Jeon SB, Lee Y, *et al.* (2015). Fermented red ginseng extract inhibits cancer cell proliferation and viability. *Journal of Medicinal Food, 18*(4), 421–428. doi:10.1089/jmf.2014.3248.

Pai M, Kuo Y, Chiang E, Tang F. (2012). S-Allylcysteine inhibits tumour progression and the epithelial–mesenchymal transition in a mouse xenograft model of oral cancer. *British Journal of Nutrition, 108*(1), 28–38. doi:10.1017/S0007114511005307.

Palozza P, Parrone N, Catalano A, Simone R. (2010). Tomato lycopene and inflammatory cascade: Basic interactions and clinical implications. *Current Medicinal Chemistry, 17,* 2547. doi:10.2174/092986710791556041.

Pannellini T, Iezzi M, Liberatore M, *et al.* (2010). A dietary tomato supplement prevents prostate cancer in TRAMP mice. *Cancer Prevention Research, 3*(10), 1284–1291.

Pashaei-Asl R, Pashaei-Asl F, Gharabaghi PM, *et al.* (2017). The inhibitory effect of ginger extract on ovarian cancer cell line: Application of systems biology. *Advanced Pharmaceutical Bulletin, 7*(2), 241–249. doi:10.15171/apb.2017.029.

Prasad S, Tyagi AK. (2015). Ginger and its constituents: Role in prevention and treatment of gastrointestinal cancer. *Gastroenterology Research and Practice, 2015,* 142979. doi:10.1155/2015/142979.

Puccinelli MT, Stan SD. (2017). Dietary bioactive diallyl trisulfide in cancer prevention and treatment. *International Journal of Molecular Sciences, 18*(8), 1645. doi:10.3390/ijms18081645.

Radhakrishnan EK, Bava SV, Narayanan SS, *et al.* (2014). [6]-Gingerol induces caspase-dependent apoptosis and prevents PMA-induced proliferation in colon cancer cells by inhibiting MAPK/AP-1 signaling. *PLoS One, 9*(8), e104401. doi:10.1371/journal.pone.0104401

Raghu R, Lu KH, Sheen LY. (2012). Recent Research progress on garlic (dà suàn) as a potential anticarcinogenic agent against major digestive cancers. *Journal of Traditional and Complementary Medicine, 2*(3), 192–201. doi:10.1016/s2225-4110(16)30099-2.

Rhode J, Fogoros S, Zick S, *et al.* (2007). Ginger inhibits cell growth and modulates angiogenic factors in ovarian cancer cells. *BMC Complementary and Alternative Medicine, 7,* 44. doi:10.1186/1472-6882-7-44.

Royston KJ, Tollefsbol TO. (2015). The epigenetic impact of cruciferous vegetables on cancer prevention. *Current Pharmacology Reports, 1*(1), 46–51. doi:10.1007/s40495-014-0003-9.

Seeram NP. (2008). Berry fruits for cancer prevention: Current status and future prospects. *Journal of Agricultural and Food Chemistry, 56*(3), 630–635. doi:10.1021/jf072504n.

Sharoni Y, Linnewiel-Hermoni K, Zango G, *et al.* (2012). The role of lycopene and its derivatives in the regulation of transcription systems: Implications for cancer prevention. *The American Journal of Clinical Nutrition, 96*(5), 1173S–1178S. doi:10.3945/ajcn.112.034645.

Shukla Y, Singh M. (2007). Cancer preventive properties of ginger a brief review. *Food and Chemical Toxicology: An International Journal Published for the British Industrial Biological Research Association, 45*(5), 683–690.

Somasagara RR, Hegde M, Chiruvella KK, Musini A, Choudhary B, Raghavan SC. (2012). Extracts of strawberry fruits induce intrinsic pathway of apoptosis in breast cancer cells and inhibits tumor progression in mice. *PLoS One, 7*(10), e47021. doi:10.1371/journal.pone.0047021.

Steinmetz KA, Kushi LH, Bostick RM, Folsom AR, Potter JD. (1994). Vegetables, fruit, and colon cancer in the Iowa Women's Health Study. *American Journal of Epidemiology, 139*(1), 1–15.

Stice CP, Xia H, Wang XD. (2018). Tomato lycopene prevention of alcoholic fatty liver disease and hepatocellular carcinoma development. *Chronic Diseases and Translational Medicine, 4*(4), 211–224. doi:10.1016/j.cdtm.2018.11.001.

Tantamango YM, Knutsen SF, Beeson WL, Fraser G, Sabate J. (2011). Foods and food groups associated with the incidence of colorectal polyps: The Adventist Health Study. *Nutrition and Cancer, 63*(4), 565–572. doi: 10.1080/01635581.2011.551988.

Traka MH, Melchini A, Coode-Bate J, *et al.* (2019). Transcriptional changes in prostate of men on active surveillance after a 12-mo glucoraphanin-rich broccoli intervention-results from the Effect of Sulforaphane on prostate CAncer PrEvention (ESCAPE) randomized controlled trial. *The American Journal of Clinical Nutrition, 109*(4), 1133–1144. doi:10.1093/ajcn/nqz012.

University College London. (2005, September 15). University College London Study Shows Beans Beat Cancer. *ScienceDaily*. Retrieved on October 22, 2019, from www.sciencedaily.com/releases/2005/09/050915002836.htm.

University Of Illinois at Urbana-Champaign. (2003, November 5). Lycopene's anti-cancer effect linked to other tomato components. *ScienceDaily*. Retrieved on October 24, 2019, from www.sciencedaily.com/releases/2003/11/031105064728.htm.

University Of Minnesota. (2003, October 29). Dietary ginger may work against cancer growth. *ScienceDaily*. Retrieved on October 24, 2019, from www.sciencedaily.com/releases/2003/10/031029064357.htm.

Wan Q, Li N, Du L, *et al.* (2019). Allium vegetable consumption and health: An umbrella review of meta-analyses of multiple health outcomes. *Food Science & Nutrition*, *7*(8), 2451–2470. doi:10.1002/fsn3.1117.

Wang CZ, Yu C, Wen XD, *et al.* (2016). American ginseng attenuates colitis-associated colon carcinogenesis in mice: Impact on gut microbiota and metabolomics. *Cancer Prevention Research (Philadelphia, PA.)*, *9*(10), 803–811. doi:10.1158/1940-6207.CAPR-15-0372.

Wang LS, Hecht SS, Carmella SG, *et al.* (2009). Anthocyanins in black raspberries prevent oesophageal tumors in rats. *Cancer Prevention Research (Philadelphia, PA.)*, *2*(1), 84–93. doi:10.1158/1940-6207.CAPR-08-0155.

Wang LS, Hecht S, Carmella S, *et al.* (2010). Berry ellagitannins may not be sufficient for prevention of tumors in the rodent esophagus. *Journal of Agricultural and Food Chemistry*, *58*(7), 3992–3995. doi:10.1021/jf9030635.

Wang TT, Schoene NW, Milner JA, Kim YS. (2012). Broccoli-derived phytochemicals indole-3-carbinol and 3,3'-diindolylmethane exerts concentration-dependent pleiotropic effects on prostate cancer cells: Comparison with other cancer preventive phytochemicals. *Molecular Carcinogenesis*, *51*(3), 244–256.

Wang Y, Jacobs EJ, Newton CC, McCullough ML. (2016). Lycopene, tomato products and prostate cancer-specific mortality among men diagnosed with nonmetastatic prostate cancer in the Cancer Prevention Study II Nutrition Cohort. *International Journal of Cancer*, *138*(12), 2846–2855.

Wong AS, Che CM, Leung KW. (2015). Recent advances in ginseng as cancer therapeutics: A functional and mechanistic overview. *Natural Product Reports*, *32*(2), 256–272. doi:10.1039/c4np00080c.

Xia H, Liu C, Li C-C, *et al.* (2018). Dietary tomato powder inhibits high-fat diet-promoted hepatocellular carcinoma with alteration of gut microbiota in mice lacking carotenoid cleavage enzymes. *Cancer Prevention Research*, *11*(12), 797–810.

Yang H, Tian T, Wu D, Guo D, Lu J. (2019). Prevention and treatment effects of edible berries for three deadly diseases: Cardiovascular disease, cancer and diabetes. *Critical Reviews in Food Science and Nutrition, 59*(12), 1903–1912.

Zhang M, Viennois E, Prasad M, *et al.* (2016). Edible ginger-derived nanoparticles: A novel therapeutic approach for the prevention and treatment of inflammatory bowel disease and colitis-associated cancer. *Biomaterials, 101,* 321–340. doi:10.1016/j.biomaterials.2016.06.018.

Zheng X, Zhou Y, Chen W, *et al.* (2018). Ginsenoside 20(S)-Rg3 prevents PKM2-targeting miR-324-5p from H19 sponging to antagonize the Warburg effect in ovarian cancer cells. *Cellular Physiology and Biochemistry: International Journal of Experimental Cellular Physiology, Biochemistry, and Pharmacology, 51*(3), 1340–1353.

Zhong XS, Ge J, Chen SW, Xiong YQ, Ma SJ, Chen Q. (2018). Association between dietary isoflavones in soy and legumes and endometrial cancer: A systematic review and meta-analysis. *Journal of the Academy of Nutrition and Dietetics, 118*(4), 637–651. doi:10.1016/j.jand.2016.09.036.

Chapter 10

The Vegetarianism Cancer Prevention Formulae: Seafood + Vegetables > Only Vegetables

The practice of abstaining from meat and other by-products of animal slaughter has been in existence since 1840. Vegetarianism has now evolved into a style of living with most of its practitioners adapting to other forms of dietary patterns. Other than health-related reasons, vegetarians attribute their motivation to religion, animal right activism, political, cultural, environmental, or aesthetic beliefs. Vegetarianism comes in a variety of forms with regards to the diet. The most common forms are semi-vegetarianism that includes infrequent eating of meat; lacto, only dairy products; ovo, eggs but not dairy products; lacto-ovo, eggs and dairy products; pescetarianism, includes fish and other seafood; and veganism, without animal flesh, dairy products, or eggs. Comparatively, the vegetarian population has a lower overall mortality rate and a reduced incidence of various noncommunicable diseases like cardiovascular diseases, inflammatory conditions, and other diet-related complications than omnivores. However, an inappropriately planned vegetarian diet puts the person at a high risk of blood-related disorders as a result of vitamin B12 deficiency among others (Figs. 1 and 2).

The association between this practice and improved health has caught the attention of the science world leading to cutting-edge research in that field. The latest is a seven-year tightly controlled study led by Michael Orlich MD, PhD, an assistant professor of preventive medicine at Loma Linda University. The study addresses the impact of vegetarian and nonvegetarian diets on colon cancer risk. Prior to this study, there was no clearly known connection between vegetarian dietary pattern and colorectal cancer risk. About half of the 77,659 adults recruited were nonvegetarians — had meat in their diets — whereas the other half were made up of four different groups of vegetarians namely: semi, lacto-ovo, pesco, and vegans.

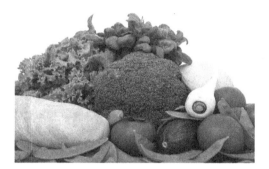

Fig. 1. Veggies

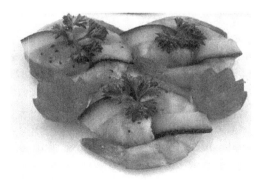

Fig. 2. Seafood with veggies

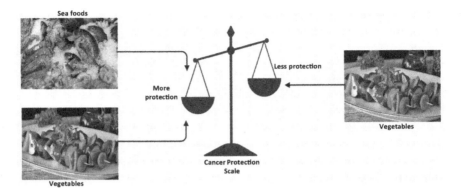

Fig. 3.   Veggies with seafood provide the most significant cancer protection

These vegetarians also had low intake of sweet, snack foods, refined grains, caloric beverages but had increased intake of fruits. Collectively, the vegetarian group averagely had a 22% reduction in the risk of developing colorectal cancer compared with the nonvegetarians. Individually, the semi-vegs, vegans, lacto-ovo, and pesco-vegetarians achieved 8%, 16%, 18%, and 43% reductions in the risk of developing colorectal cancer, respectively (Fig. 3).

Although the study provides evidence of linkage between vegetarian dietary pattern and cancer risk, there is no molecular detail to show whether the reduction is as a result of the vegetables or decreased consumption of red meat. There are, however, some works to show the protective effects of vegetables on the immune system and the consequences of excess red meat intake. The striking reduction shown by the pescetarians proves that there is more to eating vegetables alone. The inclusion of seafood especially fish plays a key role in colon protection against cancer. The dietary pattern of the semi-vegetarians presented the least protection — 8% — against colorectal cancer. It is not clearly known if the inclusion of meat in the diet attributed to this effect since the type of meat, size, and frequency of intake were not explicitly stated in the study. The study also fails to address the activities such as smoking, alcohol intake, and exercise pattern of both groups that will have a significant impact on the results. Obviously, if the vegetarian groups adapt to living a life free of alcohol and smoking and exercise frequently, an increased protection is expected compared with the nonvegetarians. A more comprehensive study is therefore needed to address these issues and also investigate the molecular linkage between the pesco-vegetarian dietary pattern and risk reduction to colorectal cancer. Also, the reduction in cancer risk should be related to other significant nutrient — vitamin B12 — deficiencies since most of these important nutrients are generally not found in vegetables.

In multiples studies, it has been demonstrated that veggies alone have a weak cancer protection; however, this protection is significantly enhanced with the addition of seafood such as fish, shrimps, and lobsters. The addition of meat provided weak to no protection against various types of cancer. These findings are suggestive that combining veggies with seafood hold the key to achieving the full chemopreventive benefits of vegetarianism. Regardless, this study provides some level of evidence of the protective effects of vegetarian diets on the colon that could be used as a preventive therapy against colorectal carcinoma. Being ranked as the fourth leading cancer in the world, colorectal cancer also ranks second in America and claims about 600,000 lives yearly. With a limited therapy, it is very prudent to institute comprehensive preventive measures of which a carefully planned pescetarian diet could be resorted to. With ultrarefined foods showing a 10% increase in cancer risk, care should be taken in maintaining a balance in our diet.

Bibliography

Appleby PN, Crowe FL, Bradbury KE, Travis RC, Key TJ. (2016). Mortality in vegetarians and comparable nonvegetarians in the United Kingdom. *The American Journal of Clinical Nutrition, 103*(1), 218–230. doi:10.3945/ ajcn.115.119461.

Dinu M, Abbate R, Gensini GF, Casini A, Sofi F. (2017). Vegetarian, vegan diets and multiple health outcomes: A systematic review with meta-analysis of observational studies. *Critical Reviews in Food Science and Nutrition, 57*(17), 3640–3649. doi:10.1080/10408398.2016.1138447.

Fiolet T, Srour B, Sellem L, *et al.* (2018). Consumption of ultra-processed foods and cancer risk: Results from NutriNet-Santé prospective cohort. *BMJ (Clinical Research Ed.), 360*, k322. doi:10.1136/bmj.k322.

Gathani T, Barnes I, Ali R, *et al.* (2017). Lifelong vegetarianism and breast cancer risk: A large multicentre case control study in India. *BMC Women's Health, 17*(1), 6. doi:10.1186/s12905-016-0357-8.

Gilsing A, Weijenberg M, Goldbohm R, Dagnelie PC, van den Brandt PA, Schouten LJ. (2016). Vegetarianism, low meat consumption and the risk of lung, postmenopausal breast and prostate cancer in a population-based cohort study. *European Journal of Clinical Nutrition, 70*, 723–729. doi:10.1038/ejcn.2016.25.

Godos J, Bella F, Sciacca S, Galvano F, Grosso G. (2016, October 6). Vegetarianism and breast, colorectal and prostate cancer risk: An overview and meta-analysis of cohort studies. *Journal of Human Nutrition and Dietetics: The Official Journal of the British Dietetic Association.* doi:10.1111/jhn.12426.

https://www.aicr.org/patients-survivors/healthy-or-harmful/vegetarian-and-vegan.html. Retrieved on October 28, 2019.

Key TJ, Appleby PN, Crowe FL, Bradbury KE, Schmidt JA, Travis RC. (2014). Cancer in British vegetarians: Updated analyses of 4998 incident cancers in a cohort of 32,491 meat eaters, 8612 fish eaters, 18,298 vegetarians, and 2246 vegans. *The American Journal of Clinical Nutrition, 100*(Suppl. 1), 378S–385S. doi:10.3945/ajcn.113.071266.

Link LB, Canchola AJ, Bernstein L, *et al.* (2013). Dietary patterns and breast cancer risk in the California Teachers Study cohort. *The American Journal of Clinical Nutrition, 98*(6), 1524–1532. doi:10.3945/ajcn.113.061184.

Orlich MJ, Singh PN, Sabaté J, *et al.* (2015). Vegetarian dietary patterns and the risk of colorectal cancers. *JAMA Internal Medicine, 175*(5), 767–776. doi:10.1001/jamainternmed.2015.59.

Sobiecki JG. (2017). Vegetarianism and colorectal cancer risk in a low-selenium environment: Effect modification by selenium status? A possible factor contributing to the null results in British vegetarians. *European Journal of Nutrition, 56*(5), 1819–1832. doi:10.1007/s00394-016-1364-0.

Tantamango-Bartley Y, Jaceldo-Siegl K, Fan J, Fraser G. (2013). Vegetarian diets and the incidence of cancer in a low-risk population. *Cancer Epidemiology, Biomarkers & Prevention: A Publication of the American Association for Cancer Research, Cosponsored by the American Society of Preventive Oncology, 22*(2), 286–294. doi:10.1158/1055-9965.EPI-12-1060.

Tantamango-Bartley Y, Knutsen SF, Knutsen R, *et al.* (2016). Are strict vegetarians protected against prostate cancer? *The American Journal of Clinical Nutrition, 103*(1), 153–160. doi:10.3945/ajcn.114.106450.

Chapter 11

The Anticancer Properties of Chocolate: More than LOVE

Chocolates and bouquets of flowers dominate the various gifts that are presented to loved ones on every 14th February. All over the world, chocolate symbolizes a true gift of love and passion regardless of the time and season; however, little or nothing is known about its health advantages associated with moderate consumption. Chocolates are derived from cocoa beans and are very rich in bioactive compounds such as flavonoids that are strong antioxidants and prevent deleterious damage to cells caused by free radicals. These damages when unchecked lead to a permanent damage of the DNA and consequently tumor growth.

At the Lombardi Comprehensive Cancer Center in Georgetown University, Robert B. Dickson, PhD, and colleagues have identified pentameric procyanidin (pentamer) — a strong antioxidant — in cocoa which has the ability to deactivate proteins involved in breast cancer proliferation, invasion, and metastasis. When these proteins are deactivated, the growth of tumor cells is hampered and restricted to its site of origin, which will ultimately increase patients' survival in real practice.

In a study led by Dr. Maria Arribas at the Science and Technology Institute of Food and Nutrition, Spain, and published in the *Molecular Nutrition and Food Research* journal, bioactive compounds discovered in cocoa prevented oxidative stress, proliferation, and induced apoptosis in animal models. There was decreased bowel cancer in rats with reduced precancerous lesions. It's been demonstrated that 35 g/day of cocoa bean has the ability to provide chemopreventive properties in colorectal cancers. In a separate study, higher intake of dry beans was significantly associated with a reduction in advanced colorectal cancer recurrence. Thus, it takes longer time for such cancers to come back in people who take higher amount of dry beans. Cocoa beans and dark chocolate have also been shown to provide protection in several cancers such as breast, prostate, ovarian, gastric, and lung cancers. Also, dark chocolate has been shown to offer health benefits in other chronic diseases such as diabetes (Fig. 1).

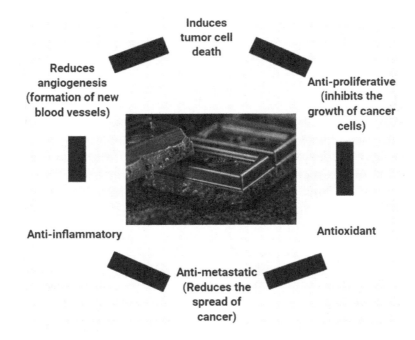

Fig. 1.   Chocolate or cocoa intake provides protection against cancer via a number of mechanisms

In the development of cancer, tumor-activating signals are triggered whereas tumor-suppressing signals are suppressed. Maintaining the fine balance between these two pathways is crucial to the development of cancer. Cocoa contains bioactive agents (polyphenols) that suppress tumor-promoting signals, thereby reducing the development of cancer. This has been shown in cancers mediated by inflammation where IL6/STAT-3 pathway was suppressed whereas programmed cell death mechanisms were promoted to kill the tumors. These effects have been demonstrated in animals as well as clinical studies involving patients. It is interesting to note that, not only does cocoa or chocolate offer direct tumor protection, but also modulate the immune system. This study is preliminary and therefore needs further investigation to substantiate these findings.

As relentless efforts are being made by cancer research scientists to unlock the code for tumorigenesis, this line of research should be embraced, encouraged, and accepted. Not all chocolates are rich in bioactive compounds that protect against inflammation, cardiovascular disorders, diabetes, and cancer; dark chocolate and cocoa powder has enormous health benefits than the milky and sweet chocolates. These studies do not confirm dark chocolate and cocoa powder as cancer preventive agents but rather, expose the potential therapeutic effects of some special bioactive agents in these products. Further rigorous experiments are needed to firmly establish the molecular mechanisms of these bioactive agents, their safe dose, and side effects if any. As it stands now, these potential therapeutics are far from human clinical trials since substantive evidence and data should be gathered at the preclinical stages to provide assurance of its safety and efficacy in humans.

Care should be taken on how chocolates are consumed as this can indirectly contribute to the growth of other cancers such as breast cancer. One ounce of dark chocolate contains 170 calories, 12 grams of fat and 24 grams of sugar while 1 ounce of cocoa powder contains 70 calories, 4 grams of fat and some trace of sugar. Although no direct link has been established, excessive consumption of chocolate can lead to overweight, which is a known contributing factor for breast cancer. Despite more light being thrown on chocolate, cocoa powder presents more health benefits due to its low fat and sugar level compared to dark chocolate.

The multifaceted nature of tumorigenesis is the greatest obstacle in cancer treatment. Moderate consumption of dark chocolate and cocoa powder will be helpful; however, positive lifestyles like exercise, smoking-free life, decreased alcohol intake, and healthy eating contribute greatly to comprehensive cancer treatment and prevention. Cancer patients should, however, not substitute their prescribed medications for chocolate since that could worsen their situation. Having an open discussion with your healthcare provider will help in making alternative decisions regarding treatments.

Bibliography

Braakhuis AJ, Campion P, Bishop KS. (2016). Reducing breast cancer recurrence: The role of dietary polyphenolics. *Nutrients, 8*(9), 547. doi:10.3390/nu8090547.

Georgetown University Medical Center. (2005, April 18). Researchers find that chocolate compound stops cancer cell cycle in lab experiments. *ScienceDaily.* Retrieved on October 28, 2019 from www.sciencedaily. com/releases/2005/04/050417213604.htm.

Hong MY, Nulton E, Shelechi M, Hernández LM, Nemoseck T. (2013). Effects of dark chocolate on azoxymethane-induced colonic aberrant crypt foci. *Nutrition and Cancer, 65*(5), 677–685. doi:10.1080/01635581. 2013.789542.

Kim J, Kim J, Shim J, Lee CY, Lee KW, Lee HJ. (2014). Cocoa phytochemicals: Recent advances in molecular mechanisms on health. *Critical Reviews in Food Science and Nutrition, 54*(11), 1458–1472. doi:10.1080/ 10408398.2011.641041.

Martin MA, Goya L, Ramos S. (2013). Potential for preventive effects of cocoa and cocoa polyphenols in cancer. *Food and Chemical Toxicology: An International Journal Published for the British Industrial Biological Research Association, 56,* 336–351. doi:10.1016/j.fct.2013.02.020.

Martín MA, Goya L, Ramos S. (2016). Preventive effects of cocoa and cocoa antioxidants in colon cancer. *Diseases (Basel, Switzerland), 4*(1), 6. doi:10.3390/diseases4010006.

Mostofsky E, Berg Johansen M, Tjønneland A, Chahal HS, Mittleman MA, Overvad K. (2017). Chocolate intake and risk of clinically apparent atrial fibrillation: The Danish Diet, Cancer, and Health Study. *Heart (British Cardiac Society), 103*(15), 1163–1167. doi:10.1136/heartjnl-2016-310357.

Pandurangan AK, Saadatdoust Z, Esa NM, Hamzah H, Ismail A. (2015). Dietary cocoa protects against colitis-associated cancer by activating the Nrf2/Keap1 pathway. *Biofactors, 41*(1), 1–14. doi:10.1002/biof.1195

Pérez-Cano FJ, Massot-Cladera M, Franch A, Castellote C, Castell M. (2013). The effects of cocoa on the immune system. *Frontiers in Pharmacology, 4*, 71. doi:10.3389/fphar.2013.00071.

Rodríguez-Ramiro I, Ramos S, López-Oliva E, *et al.* (2011). Cocoa-rich diet prevents azoxymethane-induced colonic preneoplastic lesions in rats by restraining oxidative stress and cell proliferation and inducing apoptosis. *Molecular Nutrition & Food Research, 55*, 1895–1899. doi:10.1002/mnfr.201100363.

Russo GI, Campisi D, Di Mauro M, *et al.* (2017). Dietary consumption of phenolic acids and prostate cancer: A case-control study in Sicily, Southern Italy. *Molecules (Basel, Switzerland), 22*(12), 2159. doi:10.3390/molecules22122159.

Saadatdoust Z, Pandurangan AK, Ananda Sadagopan SK, Mohd Esa N, Ismail A, Mustafa MR. (2015, December). Dietary cocoa inhibits colitis associated cancer: A crucial involvement of the IL-6/STAT3 pathway. *The Journal of Nutritional Biochemistry, 26*(12), 1547–1558. doi:10.1016/j.jnutbio.2015.07.024.

Spadafranca A, Martinez Conesa C, Sirini S, Testolin G. (2010). Effect of dark chocolate on plasma epicatechin levels, DNA resistance to oxidative stress and total antioxidant activity in healthy subjects. *British Journal of Nutrition, 103*(7), 1008–1014. doi:10.1017/S0007114509992698.

Taparia S, Khanna A. (2016). Effect of procyanidin-rich extract from natural cocoa powder on cellular viability, cell cycle progression, and chemoresistance in human epithelial ovarian carcinoma cell lines. *Pharmacognosy Magazine, 12*(Suppl. 2), S109–S115. doi:10.4103/0973-1296.182164.

Chapter 12

Physical Activity: A Crucial Factor in Reducing Cancer Risk

Physical activity involves the use of the skeletal muscles to perform a function and usually requires a lot of energy. It includes deliberate exercise in the gym, brisk walking, doing house chores, hiking, swimming, cycling, and playing soccer (Figs. 1–3). All these activities burn calories eaten from food to produce energy, a phenomenon that reduces obesity. Physical activity has health benefits such as minimizing anxiety and depression, energy production for healthy muscles and in some cases pain reduction.

In addition to the above general health benefits, a body of evidence suggests that physical activity could lower one's risk of developing cancer as well as improve the treatment of cancer patients. Physical activity has been linked to risk reduction of about 13 types of cancers including ovarian, endometrial, breast, and colon cancers. In a meta-analysis conducted in 2009, a 24% reduction in colon cancer risk was observed in participants who had an active lifestyle compared with those who were less active. In a separate analysis in 2013, 12% reduction in breast cancer risk was observed in active women compared with less active women. Active women who live

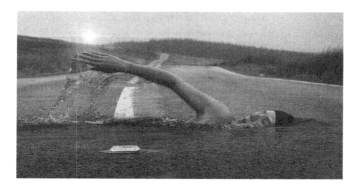

Fig. 1. Swimming

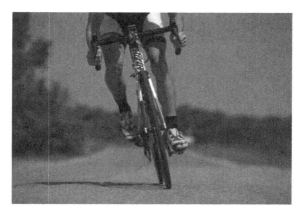

Fig. 2. Cycling

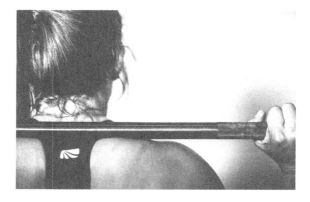

Fig. 3. Gym exercise

active lifestyles were also reported to have a 23% reduction in endo-metrial cancer compared with their less active cohorts.

The reduction in cancer risk could be as a result of decreased production of hormones and growth factors that serve as fuel or drivers for the cancer cells. Also, increase in physical activity mini-mizes inflammation, a condition that provides a favorable environment for cancer growth. Exercise also improves the immune system's function to battle any abnormal growth of cells as well as decreases the time digested food stays in the gut to prevent pro-longed exposure of carcinogens, a condition that has been described to contribute to colon cancer.

Sedentary lifestyles where an individual is less active predispose him or her to not only cancer but also other health complications such as type 2 diabetes, cardiovascular disorders, and premature deaths. Such lifestyles include lying in bed for a long time, eating late in the night, longer hours of sitting at the office or watching TV, and eating fatty/oily meals. These can lead to obesity that has been proven to be a higher risk factor for over 23 types of cancers.

One question many people ask is what is the required amount of physical activity needed to stay healthy? Although it is difficult to provide the exact amount of time, the US Department of Health and Human Services has provided a guideline that is help-ful in achieving a healthy lifestyle. Adults require at least 2 hours and 30 minutes of moderately intense physical activity per week whereas for a very intense activity, only 1 hour 15 minutes are needed. In the case of children and adolescents, at least 60 min-utes of physical activity daily is enough to provide the needed health benefit (Fig. 4).

Physical activity not only lessens cancer risk but also has a significant impact on cancer survivors. A moderate activity has been shown to lower weight gain and improve the quality of life of cancer survivors. Cancer patients who are active have been reported to have about 40–50% lower risk of recurrence and death from breast cancer. In another study, 35–49% reduction in risk of death from breast cancer was recorded in patients who were active compared with those with sedentary lifestyles. In

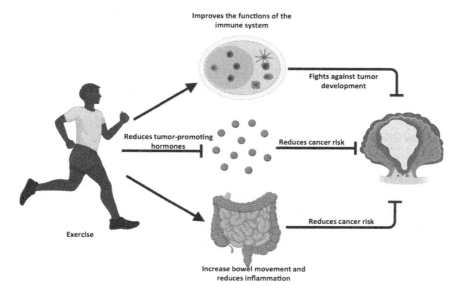

Fig. 4. Exercise strengthens the immune system and reduces tumor-promoting hormones or factors

colorectal and prostate cancers, 31% and 61% lower risk of death were recorded, respectively. These provide significant evidence that physical activity is not only a preventive measure for healthy people but could also contribute to the improvement in the overall survival of patients. It is, however, very important that patients have a well-informed discussion with their doctors on the kind of exercises to do and with which physical therapist. There are certified physical therapists who could liaise with your healthcare providers to design an effective workout plan that could be of benefit to your health.

Most of the associations with physical activity and cancer risks are correlative studies and therefore more mechanistic studies are needed to identify cause and effect. There are still other areas of research that need to be addressed such as the effect of exercise on cancer biomarkers, genetic susceptibility, drug metabolism, and the immune system. These will provide vital information that will be included in the treatment and monitoring plan of patients.

Although physical activity has great health benefits, very intense activities could be harmful to your health. Each individual should know his or her limits and pause for breaks in the middle of exercising. You can consult experts to provide help where needed to make sure you gain the maximum benefits of physical activity.

Bibliography

Ballard-Barbash, R., Friedenreich CM, Courneya KS, Siddiqi SM, McTiernan A, Alfano CM. (2012). Physical activity, biomarkers, and disease outcomes in cancer survivors: A systematic review. *Journal of the National Cancer Institute, 104*(11), 815–840.

Biswas A, Oh PI, Faulkner GE, *et al.* (2015). Sedentary time and its association with risk for disease incidence, mortality, and hospitalization in adults: A systematic review and meta-analysis. *Annals of Internal Medicine, 162*(2), 123–132.

Bonn SE, Sjölander A, Lagerros YT, *et al.* (2015). Physical activity and survival among men diagnosed with prostate cancer. *Cancer Epidemiology, Biomarkers & Prevention, 24*(1), 57–64.

Boyle T, Keegel T, Bull F, Heyworth J, Fritschi L. (2012). Physical activity and risks of proximal and distal colon cancers: A systematic review and meta-analysis. *Journal of the National Cancer Institute, 104*(20), 1548–1561.

Dowswell G, Ryan A, Taylor A, *et al.* (2012). Designing an intervention to help people with colorectal adenomas reduce their intake of red and processed meat and increase their levels of physical activity: A qualitative study. *BMC Cancer, 12*, 255. doi:10.1186/1471-2407-12-255.

Du M, Kraft P, Eliassen AH, Giovannucci E, Hankinson SE, De Vivo I. (2014). Physical activity and risk of endometrial adenocarcinoma in the Nurses' Health Study. *International Journal of Cancer, 134*(11), 2707–2716.

Eliassen AH, Hankinson SE, Rosner B, Holmes MD, Willett WC. (2010). Physical activity and risk of breast cancer among postmenopausal women. *Archives of Internal Medicine, 170*(19), 1758–1764.

Fournier A, Dos Santos G, Guillas G, *et al.* (2014). Recent recreational physical activity and breast cancer risk in postmenopausal women in the E3N cohort. *Cancer Epidemiology, Biomarkers & Prevention, 23*(9), 1893–1902.

Friedenreich C, Cust A, Lahmann PH, *et al.* (2007). Physical activity and risk of endometrial cancer: The European prospective investigation into cancer and nutrition. *International Journal of Cancer, 121*(2), 347–355.

Harriss DJ, Atkinson G, Batterham A, *et al.* (2009). Lifestyle factors and colorectal cancer risk (2): A systematic review and meta-analysis of associations with leisure-time physical activity. *Colorectal Disease: The Official Journal of the Association of Coloproctology of Great Britain and Ireland, 11*(7), 689–701. doi:10.1111/j.1463-1318.2009.01767.x.

Holick CN, Newcomb PA, Trentham-Dietz A, *et al.* (2008). Physical activity and survival after diagnosis of invasive breast cancer. *Cancer Epidemiology, Biomarkers & Prevention, 17*(2), 379–386.

Kenfield SA, Stampfer MJ, Giovannucci E, Chan JM. (2011). Physical activity and survival after prostate cancer diagnosis in the health professionals follow-up study. *Journal of Clinical Oncology, 29*(6), 726–732.

Kohler LN, Harris RB, Oren E, Roe DJ, Lance P, Jacobs ET. (2018). Adherence to nutrition and physical activity cancer prevention guidelines and development of colorectal adenoma. *Nutrients, 10*(8), 1098. doi:10.3390/nu10081098.

Lauby-Secretan B, Scoccianti C, Loomis D, *et al.* (2016). Body fatness and cancer — Viewpoint of the IARC Working Group. *New England Journal of Medicine, 375*(8), 794–798. doi:10.1056/NEJMsr1606602.

McTiernan A, Friedenreich CM, Katzmarzyk PT, *et al.* (2019). Physical activity in cancer prevention and survival: A systematic review. *Medicine and Science in Sports and Exercise, 51*(6), 1252–1261. doi:10.1249/MSS.0000000000001937.

Mishra SI, Scherer RW, Geigle PM, *et al.* (2012). Exercise interventions on health-related quality of life for cancer survivors. *The Cochrane Database of Systematic Reviews, 8*, Cd007566.

Moore SC, Lee IM, Weiderpass E, *et al.* (2016). Association of leisure-time physical activity with risk of 26 types of cancer in 1.44 million adults. *JAMA Internal Medicine, 176*(6), 816–825.

Patel AV, Friedenreich CM, Moore SC, *et al.* (2019). American college of sports medicine roundtable report on physical activity, sedentary behavior, and cancer prevention and control. *Medicine and Science in Sports and Exercise, 51*(11), 2391–2402. doi:10.1249/MSS.0000000000002117.

Robsahm TE, Aagnes B, Hjartåker A, Langseth H, Bray FI, Larsen IK. (2013). Body mass index, physical activity, and colorectal cancer by anatomical subsites: A systematic review and meta-analysis of cohort studies. *European Journal of Cancer Prevention, 22*(6), 492–505.

Rock CL, Doyle C, Demark-Wahnefried W, *et al.* (2012). Nutrition and physical activity guidelines for cancer survivors. *CA: A Cancer Journal for Clinicians, 62*(4), 243–274.

Sasazuki S, Inoue M, Shimazu T, *et al.* (2018). Development and evaluation of cancer prevention strategies in Japan, evidence-based cancer prevention recommendations for Japanese. *Japanese Journal of Clinical Oncology, 48*(6), 576–586. doi:10.1093/jjco/hyy048.

Thomson CA, McCullough ML, Wertheim BC, *et al.* (2014). Nutrition and physical activity cancer prevention guidelines, cancer risk, and mortality in the women's health initiative. *Cancer Prevention Research (Philadelphia, PA.), 7*(1), 42–53. doi:10.1158/1940-6207.CAPR-13-0258.

Wolin KY, Yan Y, Colditz GA. (2011). Physical activity and risk of colon adenoma: A meta-analysis. *British Journal of Cancer, 104*(5), 882–885.

World Cancer Research Fund/American Institute for Cancer Research. (2007). *Food, nutrition, physical activity, and the prevention of cancer: A global perspective exit disclaimer.* Washington, DC: AICR.

Wu Y, Zhang D, Kang S. (2013). Physical activity and risk of breast cancer: A meta-analysis of prospective studies. *Breast Cancer Research and Treatment, 137*(3), 869–882.

Chapter 13

NaNose: A "Nose" that Detects Early-Stage Cancer in Human Breath

With cancer mortality on ascendency, pragmatic steps have been taken to help curb this threat. Despite the numerous arrays of diagnostic techniques developed, early detection of cancer is still a battle faced by clinicians and researchers. Early detection of cancer helps to improve cancer treatment and patient survival. Plasma gelsolin in the blood has shown promise in detecting ovarian cancer at an early stage as well as predicting how successful a surgery will be. This comes as great news since ovarian cancer is mostly detected at late stages with difficulty in treatment. Regardless, more efforts are needed in producing reliable early detection platforms to maximize diagnosis and effective treatments. Beside using less-invasive approaches, it will be interesting to further explore noninvasive (without using needles/surgical instruments) techniques that will make early diagnosis quicker, more convenient, and cheaper.

Stomach cancer is also diagnosed in the late stage and hence very difficult to treat. Popularly known as the cancer of the aged — since about two-thirds of the cases are reported in people above

65 years — stomach cancer affects 7,300 people in the United Kingdom. This uncommon cancer is mostly seen among people with *Helicobacter pylori* infection, men, stomach inflammation victims, those eating lots of salted, smoked, or pickled foods, people who smoke cigarette and those who have a family history of stomach cancer. Endoscopy has been the most widely used diagnostic technique for stomach cancer; however, its ability to detect the early stages of the cancer is limited. Regardless of the number of biomarkers discovered, stomach cancer still presents as a predominantly late-stage disease and is very difficult to treat. This has become the motivation of numerous studies to find noninvasive approaches to curbing the situation.

Hossam Haick, PhD, head of the laboratory for nanomaterial-based device and volatile biomarkers, Technion — Israel Institute of Technology, Haifa, has developed a breath technique, NaNose, that uses exhaled air to detect the earliest signs of stomach cancer. This is a noninvasive test that efficiently and accurately detects changes in the compounds of the exhaled air that signal cancer development (Fig. 1). NaNose uses a nanoarray technique where a set of atoms are analyzed from the exhaled air using a computer to detect some specific compounds that have a link to stomach cancer. Cancer produces volatile organic compounds (VOCs) that evaporate with exhaled air giving a unique scent, which can serve as a "blue print" for that particular cancer. In the study, two different breath samples were collected from the 484 participants that were recruited. In total 99 out of the 484 subjects were diagnosed of stomach cancer; their alcohol intake and smoking habits as well as *H. pylori* infection detection were taken into account during the study.

The first sample collected was analyzed with gas chromatography mass spectrometry (GCMS) that measures the different organic compounds while the second sample was analyzed with Dr. Haick's NaNose. The nanoarray technique provided a more accurate and robust distinction of the different stages in stomach cancer development. NaNose gave a greater than 80% accurate diagnosis of cases and was able to grade subjects into low risk and high risk. "Currently, there is no perfect noninvasive tool to screen for stomach cancer," Haick said. "Small and inexpensive sensing

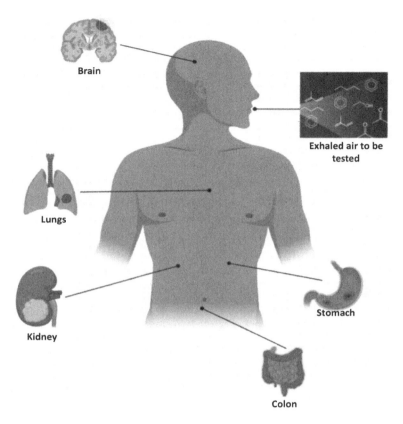

Fig. 1. Mechanized circuits termed as "noses" can detect early-stage cancers by "sniffing" human breath and other body fluids

technology could be developed and used to fulfil these clinical needs," he also added.

NaNose presents a more affordable, accurate, efficient, and robust means of diagnosing early-stage cancers and this technology will also be beneficial in other chronic and life-threatening diseases such as diabetes, hypertension, and other inflammatory diseases. NaNose will be a blessing to the developing world since the standard gastric cancer detection using GCMS is more expensive and takes time. The NaNose technology should be installed in mobile devices or most handheld devices as a software application that could be easily used by the public in their daily activities. This will help reveal early stages of diseases and will inform the necessary treatment before they become more complicated and aggressive. Regardless of the promising diagnostic effects of NaNose, larger trials are needed to provide more convincing data to support and affirm the initial findings. The research world awaits results from the large trial underway in Europe in the coming months. Notwithstanding, the noninvasiveness, fast speed, affordability, and accurate diagnostic precisions exhibited by NaNose demand massive attention especially in the area of early-stage detection of cancer.

Using commercial electronic noses, exhaled breath and urine samples have been analyzed and provided promising results in the early detection of breast cancer. With test accuracies of 95.2% and 85% for two different electronic noses used, these platforms present as convenient diagnostic candidates to revolutionize early cancer detection. In addition to electronic noses, electrocardiogram has been implicated in the detection of ovarian, breast, prostate, colon, gastric, esophageal, and hematological malignancies.

In the detection of aggressive cancers that affect the prostate, using electronic nose provided sensitivity and specificity of 71.4% and 92.6%, respectively. This was also demonstrated in another study where sensitivity and specificity were 78% and 67%, respectively. In distinguishing lung cancer patients from healthy cohorts, e-nose provided test accuracies of 83% and 86% in two separate analyses. Greater than 80% test accuracies have also been shown in head-and-neck squamous cell, colorectal, and bladder cancers. With test accuracy greater than 80%, e-nose was able to differentiate head-and-neck cancers from other types of cancers such as bladder and colon cancers. Beside the detection of cancers via less-invasive and noninvasive approaches, e-nose has been shown to detect genetic mutations (EGFR) in lung cancer patients. When this is developed further, it could be helpful in providing targeted therapies to patients presenting such mutations. This mutation has been shown to be present in lots of cancers. E-nose also has a very high prediction rate to nonresponders of immunotherapy (anti-PD1) in non-small cell lung cancer (NSCLC). This could potentially help prevent administering certain kinds of immunotherapies to patients who are likely not to respond, an intervention that will prevent unwanted side effects and also provide alternative treatment strategies to improve patients' survival. Although the above findings are interesting and promising, more clinical studies are needed to warrant their application in the clinics. This will enable detection and provide resolutions to limitations that might come with this new technology.

Machine-learning analysis of nanoresolution images of cell surfaces also provides 94% test accuracy in bladder cancer detection. Urine samples are collected from patients and floating cells isolated for imaging and analysis. This noninvasive approach provides significant improvement compared with the conventional means of detecting bladder cancer. Gradually, early detection of cancer is moving away from being invasive to less-invasive and then noninvasive. With technological advancement, this transition seeks to improve the turnaround time and robustness as well as affordability. If carefully managed, machine learning or artificial intelligence will emerge as the biggest game changer in cancer diagnosis and treatment.

Bibliography

Asare-Werehene M, Communal L, Carmona E, *et al.* (2019). Pre-operative circulating plasma gelsolin predicts residual disease and detects early stage ovarian cancer. *Scientific Reports, 9*(1), 13924. doi:10.1038/s41598-019-50436-1.

Asimakopoulos AD, Del Fabbro D, Miano R, *et al.* (2014). Prostate cancer diagnosis through electronic nose in the urine headspace setting: A pilot study. *Prostate Cancer and Prostatic Diseases, 17*(2), 206–211. doi:10.1038/pcan.2014.11.

de Vries R, Muller M, van der Noort V, *et al.* (2019). Prediction of response to anti-PD-1 therapy in patients with non-small-cell lung cancer by electronic nose analysis of exhaled breath. *Annals of Oncology, 30*(10), 1660–1666. doi:10.1093/annonc/mdz279.

Heers H, Gut JM, Hegele A, *et al.* (2018). Non-invasive detection of bladder tumors through volatile organic compounds: A pilot study with an electronic nose. *Anticancer Research, 38*(2), 833–837.

Herman-Saffar O, Boger Z, Libson S, Lieberman D, Gonen R, Zeiri Y. (2018). Early non-invasive detection of breast cancer using exhaled breath and urine analysis. *Computers in Biology and Medicine, 96*, 227–232. doi:10.1016/j.compbiomed.2018.04.002.

Kort S, Brusse-Keizer M, Gerritsen JW, van der Palen J. (2017). Data analysis of electronic nose technology in lung cancer: Generating prediction models by means of Aethena. *Journal of Breath Research.* doi:10.1088/1752-7163/aa6b08.

Leunis N, Boumans ML, Kremer B, *et al.* (2014). Application of an electronic nose in the diagnosis of head and neck cancer. *Laryngoscope, 124*(6), 1377–1381. doi:10.1002/lary.24463.

McWilliams A, Beigi P, Srinidhi A, Lam S, MacAulay CE. (2015). Sex and smoking status effects on the early detection of early lung cancer in high-risk smokers using an electronic nose. *IEEE Transactions on Bio-Medical Engineering, 62*(8), 2044–2054. doi:10.1109/TBME.2015.2409092.

Nakhleh MK, Amal H, Jeries R, *et al.* (2017). Diagnosis and classification of 17 diseases from 1404 subjects via pattern analysis of exhaled molecules. *ACS Nano, 11*(1), 112–125. doi:10.1021/acsnano.6b04930.

Omura Y, Lu D, O'Young B, *et al.* (2015). New non-invasive safe, quick, economical method of detecting various cancers was found using QRS complex or rising part of T-wave of recorded ECGs. Cancers can be screened along with their biochemical parameters & therapeutic effects of any cancer treatments can be evaluated using recorded ECGs of the same individual. *Acupuncture & Electro-Therapeutics Research, 40*(1), 1–15.

Roine A, Veskimäe E, Tuokko A, *et al.* (2014). Detection of prostate cancer by an electronic nose: A proof of principle study. *The Journal of Urology, 192*(1), 230–234. doi:10.1016/j.juro.2014.01.113.

Santini G, Mores N, Penas A, *et al.* (2016). Electronic nose and exhaled breath NMR-based metabolomics applications in airways disease. *Current Topics in Medicinal Chemistry, 16*(14), 1610–1630.

Shlomi D, Abud M, Liran O, *et al.* (2017). Detection of lung cancer and EGFR mutation by electronic nose system. *Journal of Thoracic Oncology: Official Publication of the International Association for the Study of Lung Cancer.* doi:10.1016/j.jtho.2017.06.073.

Sokolov I, Dokukin ME, Kalaparthi V, *et al.* (2018). Noninvasive diagnostic imaging using machine-learning analysis of nanoresolution images of cell surfaces: Detection of bladder cancer. *Proceedings of the National*

Academy of Sciences of the United States of America, 115(51), 12920–12925. doi:10.1073/pnas.1816459115.

Tirzīte M, Bukovskis M, Strazda G, Jurka N, Taivans I. (2017). Detection of lung cancer in exhaled breath with electronic nose using support vector machine analysis. *Journal of Breath Research, 11*: 036009. doi:10.1088/1752-7163/aa7799.

van de Goor RM, Leunis N, van Hooren MR, *et al.* (2017). Feasibility of electronic nose technology for discriminating between head and neck, bladder, and colon carcinomas. *European Archives of Oto-Rhino-Laryngology: Official Journal of the European Federation of Oto-Rhino-Laryngological Societies (EUFOS): Affiliated with the German Society for Oto-Rhino-Laryngology — Head and Neck Surgery, 274*(2), 1053–1060. doi:10.1007/s00405-016-4320-y.

van de Goor R, Hardy J, van Hooren M, Kremer B, Kross KW. (2019). Detecting recurrent head and neck cancer using electronic nose technology: A feasibility study. *Head & Neck, 41*(9), 2983–2990. doi:10.1002/hed.25787.

van de Goor R, van Hooren M, Dingemans AM, Kremer B, Kross K. (2018). Training and validating a portable electronic nose for lung cancer screening. *Journal of Thoracic Oncology: Official Publication of the International Association for the Study of Lung Cancer, 13*, 676–681. doi:10.1016/j.jtho.2018.01.024.

Westenbrink E, Arasaradnam RP, O'Connell N, *et al.* (2015). Development and application of a new electronic nose instrument for the detection of colorectal cancer. *Biosensors & Bioelectronics, 67*, 733–738. doi:10.1016/j.bios.2014.10.044.

Chapter 14

Cancer Myths and Misconceptions

Being one of the most deadly diseases on the globe, cancer has caused a huge panic both in the developed and developing nations. With a continuous rise in newly diagnosed cases and mortality rate, the cancer research community has generated a battery of treatment options to assuage this condition. Despite the great effort exhibited by researchers to curb this canker, cancer continues to claim lives and render many victims incapacitated. These reasons have prompted many people to associate cancer with some misconceptions that deceive the general public. Here, I carefully discuss some of the common myths that have been linked to cancer for many years.

Do Cosmetics/Toiletries Cause Cancer?

Shampoos, lipsticks, deodorants, toothpastes, hair dyes, talcum powder, and moisturizers are all considered to be part of this group (Fig. 1). There have been a link associated with these products and cancer; however, there is NO clear evidence that supports this link. Studies have been done on chemicals in cosmetics such

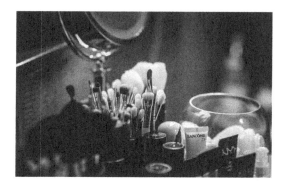

Fig. 1. Cosmetics

as coal tar, titanium dioxide nanoparticles, hyaluronic acid, octocrylene, and aluminum; however, no concrete causal link has been established.

There are various concerns whether or not the chemicals in these products could increase cancer risk. In most parts of the world, there are very strict regulations on the use of cancer-causing chemicals in the manufacturing of these products. This serves as a check on the safety of cosmetics and toiletries sold to the general public. In a hoax email, deodorant is said to increase the risk of breast cancer since it blocks the holes in the skin and prevents sweating, leading to the accumulation of a toxin in the lymph glands under the armpit. The body has several means of clearing toxins — sweating is one. Also, breast cancer originates from the breast tissues and then migrates to the lymph glands but not vice versa. The blocking of sweating pores cannot cause breast cancer and there is also NO scientifically proven study confirming the link between cosmetics and cancer risk.

There have been some occasions where talcum powder has been called off the market for suspicion of increasing cancer risk. This is because at its natural state, talc may contain asbestos, a cancer-causing agent. It was once detected that using talcum powder on genitals could increase ovarian cancer risk by 33% as reported in the journal *Epidemiology*. Although no scientific study has been done to establish causality, the American Cancer Society has advised that individuals should either avoid or limit the use of cosmetics containing talc. In 2018, Health Canada announced that products containing talc might pose a health risk to individuals. Specifically, they mentioned that inhaling talc powder could cause lung damage as well as ovarian cancer when put on the female genitalia. These health damages have resulted in lawsuits involving one of the biggest cosmetic manufacturers, Johnson & Johnson, where over $4.7 billion were paid to 22 women. Although correlative evidence is available to link the use of cosmetics to cancer development, substantial mechanistic evidence is needed to establish causality. Health regulatory bodies around the world are on the lookout to efficiently scrutinize all products released into the market for human use. Regardless, there have been a few studies that claim longer exposure to cosmetic chemicals might lead to the development of cancer such as ovarian and endometrial cancers.

Do Artificial Sweeteners Cause Cancer?

No. There is no conclusive evidence to support the link between artificial sweeteners and cancer risk. Safety studies have been conducted on saccharin, neotame, aspartame, sucralose, and cyclamate among others and no cancer-causing agent has been shown (Fig. 2). With the exception of cyclamate, all the other

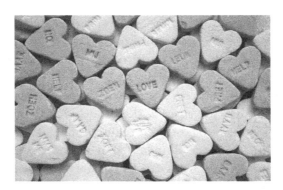

Fig. 2.   Artificial sweeteners

artificial sweeteners have been approved by the FDA to be sold on the American market. However, artificial sweeteners should be taken in moderation since higher intake has been associated with possible risk of developing cancer. Although dietary artificial sweeteners have a weak association with cancer risk, soft drinks sweetened with artificial sugars have been shown to be associated with increased risk of cancers such as colon, breast, and gastric cancers.

Is Cancer Contagious?

To a large extent NO. In general, cancer cannot be transferred from one person to another. However, in organ or tissue transplants, there is an increased risk of transplant-associated cancer if the donor has a past history of cancer, which usually occurs in 2 out of every 10,000 transplant cases. Surgeons usually avoid organs or tissues from donors with cancer to prevent future complications. Also, some bacteria (*Helicobacter pylori*) and viruses (such as human papillomavirus, HPV) are highly associated with cancer, hence catching the infection from someone could possibly increase your risk of developing some types of cancers. Although cancer is not contagious, care should be taken during organ transplant and viral/ bacterial infections (Fig. 3).

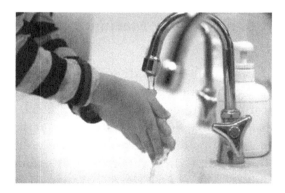

Fig. 3. Handwashing to prevent disease transmission

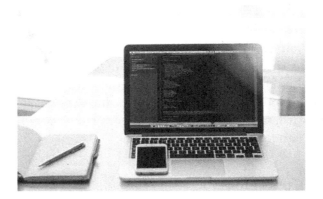

Fig. 4.   Electronics

Mobiles Phones, Power Lines, Wi-Fi, Bluetooth, and Microwaves Have Been Linked with Cancer

This is not entirely true. These devices emit low-energy nonionizing radiation that cannot change or alter the genetic makeup of our cells. Various studies have been conducted with the aim of establishing a strong link between these devices and cancer; however, there is not enough evidence to confirm this link. Although no causal link has been established, care should be taken when using gadgets that emit radiations since it could be harmful to your health but not necessarily cause cancer (Fig. 4).

Do X-ray and Body Imaging Machines Increase Cancer Risk?

X-ray and CT scan machines provide great health screening benefits to patients. Notwithstanding, they use high-energy ionizing radiation that can alter the genetic makeup of a cell to cause cancer. Experts, however, manage to decrease the radiation dose in order to minimize any possible harm. Also, the area of the body, age, and gender determine the level of risk. For example, radiation at the chest region is more dangerous compared to that of the

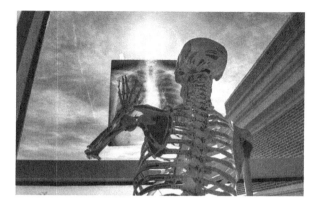

Fig. 5. Radiations

pelvic area; babies and young patients also stand a very high risk, likewise females. Various health protection agencies have been established across the world to make sure patients receive a safe dose. However, when an individual is exposed to higher levels of radiations over time, there is a greater probability that genetic alterations could occur, increasing the risk of developing cancer (Fig. 5).

Is There a Link Between Plastic Bottles/Containers and Cancer?

Circulating hoax emails warn the public against reusing plastic bottles, freezing water in them, and microwaving food in plastic containers (Fig. 6). Their reason is that, such practices lead to the release of dioxin and DEHA from the plastic that can cause cancer in users. The WHO's International Agency for Research on Cancer and US Environmental Protection Agency state that there hasn't been any convincing scientific evidence to substantiate these health warnings against plastic use.

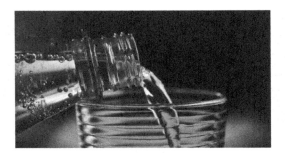

Fig. 6.   Plastics

Are Hair Dyes Safe?

Hair dyes are very popular these days and are patronized by both women and men, although the patronage is done more by women. Hair dyes come in different types. There are temporary, semi-permanent, and permanent hair dyes on the market. The huge patronage of hair dyes and the exposure of skin to the chemicals have caused lots of questions to be asked on whether the usage is associated with cancer development. There are several studies conducted on the link between hair dyes and cancer risk; however, all of these are epidemiological and do not establish any mechanistic link. Other than this, there are reports that indicate an association between hair dye application and increased risk of blood and bone marrow cancers. In the case of bladder and breast cancers, conflicting reports have emerged as some report no association whereas others report an association. Altogether, there have not been lots of mechanistic studies to nail it down as to whether hair dye application is linked with cancer development. Nonetheless, hair dyes should be used with care since their risk of developing cancer is hugely dependent on the chemicals (Fig. 7).

Conclusion

Most of these misconceptions are started by hoax emails that flood our inbox. The general public is therefore warned against such

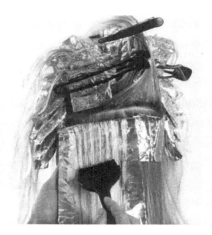

Fig. 7. Hair dye

emails and are entreated to inquire from their local cancer societies or foundations for explanations when in doubt.

Bibliography

Andrew AS, Schned AR, Heaney JA, Karagas MR. (2004). Bladder cancer risk and personal hair dye use. *International Journal of Cancer, 109*(4), 581–586.

Bosetti C, Gallus S, Talamini R, *et al.* (2009). Artificial sweeteners and the risk of gastric, pancreatic, and endometrial cancers in Italy. *Cancer Epidemiology, Biomarkers & Prevention: A Publication of the American Association for Cancer Research, Cosponsored by the American Society of Preventive Oncology, 18*(8), 2235–2238. doi:10.1158/1055-9965.EPI-09-0365.

Bukhari SNA, Roswandi NL, Waqas M, *et al.* (2018). Hyaluronic acid, a promising skin rejuvenating biomedicine: A review of recent updates and pre-clinical and clinical investigations on cosmetic and nutricosmetic effects. *International Journal of Biological Macromolecules, 120:* 1682–1695. doi:10.1016/j.ijbiomac.2018.09.188.

Cosmetic Ingredient Review Expert Panel. (2008). Final safety assessment of coal tar as used in cosmetics. *International Journal of Toxicology, 27*(Suppl. 2), 1–24. doi:10.1080/10915810802244405.

Cramer DW, Vitonis AF, Terry KL, Welch WR, Titus LJ. (2016). The association between talc use and ovarian cancer: A retrospective case-control study in two US states. *Epidemiology (Cambridge, Mass.)*, *27*(3), 334–346. doi:10.1097/EDE.0000000000000434.

Darbre PD. (2005). Aluminium, antiperspirants and breast cancer. *Journal of Inorganic Biochemistry*, *99*(9), 1912–1919. doi:10.1016/j.jinorg-bio.2005.06.001.

Hodge A, Bassett J, Milne R, English D, Giles G. (2018). Consumption of sugar-sweetened and artificially sweetened soft drinks and risk of obesity-related cancers. *Public Health Nutrition*, *21*(9), 1618–1626. doi:10.1017/S1368980017002555.

Hoover RN, Strasser PH. (1980). Artificial sweeteners and human bladder cancer. Preliminary results. *Lancet*, *1*(8173), 837–840.

Howe GR, Burch JD, Miller AB, *et al.* (1977). Artificial sweeteners and human bladder cancer. *Lancet*, *2*(8038), 578–581.

https://globalnews.ca/news/4732199/talcum-powder-ovarian-cancer/. Retrieved on October 29, 2019.

https://www.cancer.gov/about-cancer/causes-prevention/risk/diet/artificial-sweeteners-fact-sheet. Retrieved on October 29, 2019.

https://www.cancer.gov/about-cancer/causes-prevention/risk/myths. Retrieved on October 29, 2019.

https://www.cancer.org/cancer/cancer-causes/talcum-powder-and-cancer.html. Retrieved on October 29, 2019.

Huncharek M, Kupelnick B. (2005). Personal use of hair dyes and the risk of bladder cancer: Results of a meta-analysis. *Public Health Reports*, *120*(1), 31–38.

John EM, McGuire V, Thomas D, *et al.* (2013). Diagnostic chest X-rays and breast cancer risk before age 50 years for BRCA1 and BRCA2 mutation carriers. *Cancer Epidemiology, Biomarkers & Prevention: A Publication of the American Association for Cancer Research, Cosponsored by the American Society of Preventive Oncology*, *22*(9), 1547–1556. doi:10.1158/1055-9965.EPI-13-0189.

Komori S, Ito Y, Nakamura Y, *et al.* (2008). A long-term user of cosmetic cream containing estrogen developed breast cancer and endometrial hyperplasia. *Menopause*, *15*(6), 1191–1192. doi:10.1097/gme.0b013e318172847d.

Koutros S, Silverman DT, Baris D, *et al.* (2011). Hair dye use and risk of bladder cancer in the New England bladder cancer study. *International Journal of Cancer*, *129*(12), 2894–904.

Maipas S, Nicolopoulou-Stamati P. (2015). Sun lotion chemicals as endocrine disruptors. *Hormones (Athens)*, *14*(1), 32–46.

Mendelsohn JB, Li QZ, Ji BT, *et al.* (2009). Personal use of hair dye and cancer risk in a prospective cohort of Chinese women. *Cancer Science, 100*(6), 1088–1091.

Mishra A, Ahmed K, Froghi S, Dasgupta P. (2015). Systematic review of the relationship between artificial sweetener consumption and cancer in humans: Analysis of 599,741 participants. *International Journal of Clinical Practice, 69*(12), 1418–1426. doi:10.1111/ijcp.12703.

Morrison AS, Buring JE. (1980). Artificial sweeteners and cancer of the lower urinary tract. *The New England Journal of Medicine, 302*(10), 537–541. doi:10.1056/NEJM198003063021001.

Ros MM, Gago-Dominguez M, Aben KK, et al. (2012). Personal hair dye use and the risk of bladder cancer: A case-control study from The Netherlands. *Cancer Causes and Control, 23*(7), 1139–1148.

Schernhammer ES, Bertrand KA, Birmann BM, Sampson L, Willett WC, Feskanich D. (2012). Consumption of artificial sweetener- and sugar-containing soda and risk of lymphoma and leukemia in men and women. *The American Journal of Clinical Nutrition, 96*(6), 1419–1428. doi:10.3945/ajcn.111.030833.

Takkouche B, Etminan M, Montes-Martinez A. (2005). Personal use of hair dyes and risk of cancer: A meta-analysis. *JAMA: The Journal of the American Medical Association, 293*(20), 2516–2525.

van Eyk AD. (2015). The effect of five artificial sweeteners on Caco-2, HT-29 and HEK-293 cells. *Drug and Chemical Toxicology, 38*(3), 318–327. doi:10.3109/01480545.2014.966381.

Wynder EL, Stellman, SD. (1980, March 14). Artificial sweetener use and bladder cancer: A case-control study. *Science, 207*(4436), 1214–1216.

Zhang Y, de Sanjose S, Bracci PM, *et al.* (2008). Personal use of hair dye and the risk of certain subtypes of non-Hodgkin lymphoma. *American Journal of Epidemiology, 167*(11), 1321–1331.

Chapter 15

"Sensible Use" of the Sun Can Heal

Sunlight has mostly been demonized for causing most medically related complications including cancer. The presence of ultraviolet (UV) light from the sun has been implicated in the risk of melanoma and basal and squamous cell skin cancers. This has been attributed to the increased exposure of the body to sunlight (UVB). There are two different types of UV wavelengths: UVA and UVB. UVB is considered to be the healthy wavelength while the UVA is known for its deleterious effects on the skin due to its high penetration power. In 1915, Hoffman first showed the association between sunlight and cancer risk where he reported mortality from cancer at various latitudes in different cities. Since then, there have been several documented reports advancing this field of research (Fig. 1).

Despite these purported demonized effects of the sun, another field of research has exploited its therapeutic potencies through the manufacturing of vitamin D against cancer. UVB is a major contributor for the synthesis of vitamin D by the body. This healthy wavelength is very high during the midday but low in the mornings and evenings. Thus, a decrease in "sensible" sunlight exposure may lead to decreased vitamin D production and hence increased risk of

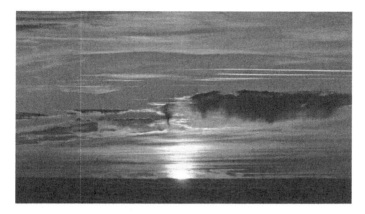

Fig. 1. Sunrise

cancer especially melanoma — a deadly skin cancer. In the Daily Mail, Prof. Angus Dalgleish reported, *"Research shows that a large percentage of people in the UK are deficient in vitamin D partly because we can't make any from the sun for about six months of the year ... I'd like to see all other cancer units automatically checking their patients' blood levels. It's cheap and quick and I guarantee they would be amazed at just how low many were."*

Researchers at the department of family medicine and public health, University of California, San Diego have reported a study after reviewing information from more than 100 countries about the association between sunlight and prostate cancer risk. They recorded a high risk of pancreatic cancer for people living in places with low sunlight leading to decreased synthesis of vitamin D. Dr. Cedric Garland, a coauthor and Adjunct Professor with the university added, *"If you're living at a high latitude or in a place with a lot of heavy cloud cover, you can't make vitamin D most of the year, which results in a higher-than-normal risk of getting pancreatic cancer. People who live in sunny countries near the equator have only one-sixth of the age-adjusted incidence rate of pancreatic cancer as those who live far from it. The importance of sunlight deficiency strongly suggests — but does not prove — that vitamin D deficiency may contribute to risk of pancreatic cancer."* A similar finding has also been reported by Rosso and colleagues at the

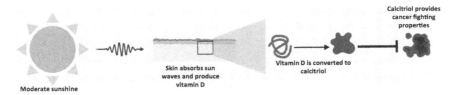

Fig. 2.   Moderate exposure to sunlight results in vitamin D synthesis that provides a cancer-fighting advantage

Cancer Prevention Centre, Turin, Italy where a population-based case control study revealed increased survival rate for melanoma patients who had adequate exposure to the sun prior to diagnosis (Fig. 2).

These findings suggest that, sunlight in itself has no direct therapeutic effect on cancer but rather drives the synthesis of vitamin D which in turn does the magic. The sun is not the only drive for vitamin D synthesis since other foods like salmon, tuna, orange juice, milk, and egg yolk, among others, provide natural source for this essential vitamin. However, the amount of vitamin D needed by the body cannot solely be provided by such foods hence the need for sensible exposure to the sun. As one of the oldest steroid hormones, vitamin D has receptors in almost every cell in the body. Generally, vitamin D when synthesized is converted into calcitriol — an activated form — which provides the following anticancer properties:

1. Increase apoptosis (programmed cell death) of mutated cells which have the tendency of evolving into cancer cells
2. Reduce angiogenesis (synthesis of new blood vessels) which decreases the spread and intensity of the cancer cells

A vitamin D expert, Dr. William Grant, PhD, has reported that about two million cancer deaths worldwide could be prevented each year with higher levels of vitamin D. Despite the protective effects of vitamin D, care should be taken in their use. Moderation is the key since excessive dose could result in hypervitaminosis D, a condition where there is increased calcium concentration in the blood that leads to over calcification of bones, kidney, heart, and other soft tissues.

It is therefore advised to adhere to the moderate exposure of the body to sunlight especially the UVB, which is very high during the midday. The intake of vegetables and fruits is highly recommended to provide high antioxidants against free radicals that are produced during sun burn. The use of sunscreens could also protect your body from sunlight that could lead to decreased vitamin D synthesis and increased risk of cancer. Take advantage of the sun, sensibly expose larger part of the body at the right time, eat vegetables and fruits in moderation, and enjoy good protection against cancer risk. It will also be of great benefit if more clinical studies are conducted to provide substantial evidence of the protection of sensible sunlight exposure or vitamin against cancer. As to whether sunlight exposure in different parts of the world might influence the level of protection, this is yet to be investigated.

Bibliography

Deeb KK, Trump DL, Johnson CS. (2007). Vitamin D signaling pathways in cancer: Potential for anticancer therapeutics. *Nature Reviews Cancer,* *7*(9), 684–700.

Engel LS, Satagopan J, Sima CS, *et al.* (2014). Sun exposure, vitamin D receptor genetic variants, and risk of breast cancer in the Agricultural Health Study. *Environmental Health Perspectives,* *122*(2), 165–171. doi:10.1289/ehp.1206274.

Freedman DM, Cahoon EK, Rajaraman P, *et al.* (2013). Sunlight and other determinants of circulating 25-hydroxyvitamin D levels in black and white participants in a nationwide U.S. study. *American Journal of Epidemiology,* *177*(2), 180–192. doi:10.1093/aje/kws223.

Garland CF, Cuomo RE, Gorham ED, Zeng K, Mohr SB. (2015). Cloud cover-adjusted ultraviolet B irradiance and pancreatic cancer incidence in 172 countries. *The Journal of Steroid Biochemistry and Molecular Biology,* *155*, 257–263. doi:10.1016/j.jsbmb.2015.04.004.

He Y, Timofeeva M, Farrington SM, *et al.* (2018). Exploring causality in the association between circulating 25-hydroxyvitamin D and colorectal cancer risk: A large Mendelian randomisation study. *BMC Medicine,* *16*(1), 142. doi:10.1186/s12916-018-1119-2.

Holt PR, Arber N, Halmos B, *et al.* (2002). Colonic epithelial cell proliferation decreases with increasing levels of serum 25-hydroxy vitamin D. *Cancer Epidemiology, Biomarkers, and Prevention, 11*(1), 113–119.

https://www.dailymail.co.uk/health/article-1390243/Sun-CAN-protect-skin-cancer.html. Retrieved on October 29, 2019.

International Agency for Research on Cancer Working Group on artificial ultraviolet (UV) light and skin cancer. (2007). The association of use of sunbeds with cutaneous malignant melanoma and other skin cancers: A systematic review. *International Journal of Cancer, 120*(5), 1116–1122. doi:10.1002/ijc.22453.

Karami S, Colt JS, Stewart PA, *et al.* (2016). A case-control study of occupational sunlight exposure and renal cancer risk. *International Journal of Cancer, 138*(7), 1626–1633. doi:10.1002/ijc.29902.

Ma Y, Zhang P, Wang F, *et al.* (2011). Association between vitamin D and risk of colorectal cancer: A systematic review of prospective studies. *Journal of Clinical Oncology, 29*(28), 3775–3782.

Moukayed M, Grant WB. (2017). The roles of UVB and vitamin D in reducing risk of cancer incidence and mortality: A review of the epidemiology, clinical trials, and mechanisms. *Reviews in Endocrine & Metabolic Disorders.* doi:10.1007/s11154-017-9415-2.

Rosso S, Sera F, Segnan N, Zanetti R. (2008). Sun exposure prior to diagnosis is associated with improved survival in melanoma patients: Results from a long-term follow-up study of Italian patients. *European Journal of Cancer, 44*(9), 1275–1281. doi:10.1016/j.ejca.2008.03.009.

Schuch AP, Moreno NC, Schuch NJ, Menck CFM, Garcia CCM. (2017). Sunlight damage to cellular DNA: Focus on oxidatively generated lesions. *Free Radical Biology & Medicine, 107*, 110–124. doi:10.1016/j.freeradbiomed.2017.01.029.

Surdu S, Fitzgeraldab EF, Bloom MS, *et al.* (2014). Polymorphisms in DNA repair genes XRCC1 and XRCC3, occupational exposure to arsenic and sunlight, and the risk of non-melanoma skin cancer in a European case-control study. *Environmental Research, 134*, 382–389. doi:10.1016/j.envres.2014.08.020.

Vallès X, Alonso MH, López-Caleya JF, *et al.* (2018). Colorectal cancer, sun exposure and dietary vitamin D and calcium intake in the MCC-Spain study. *Environment International, 121*(Pt 1), 428–434. doi:10.1016/j.envint.2018.09.030.

Chapter 16

Big Headed People at Risk of Cancer

The drastic surge in newly diagnosed cancer cases has prompted research and clinical scientists to investigate other possible means of cancer risks in order to improve diagnostic efficiency and treatment modalities. A new area of cancer research gaining popularity is the association between cancer and physical traits such as height, weight, eye color, and hair color. Although a positive link has been established with these traits, further research studies are needed to confirm these connections. Another surprising revelation is the association between head circumference and cancer risk.

Charis Eng, the lead researcher at the Genomic Medicine Institute, Cleveland Clinic, has conducted a study into this association and showed a positive correlation of increased head circumference and cancer risk. The 127 patients screened carried a genetic mutation that causes Cowden syndrome — a rare autosomal dominant inherited disorder characterized by multiple tumor-like growths — associated with increased head size and cancer risk. Big head was defined as head circumference greater than 58 cm for men and 57 cm for women. The study revealed that 75% of the patients with Cowden syndrome had a large head and an

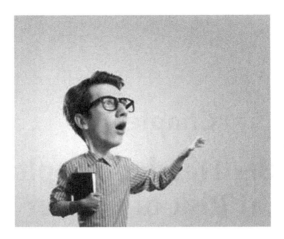

Fig. 1.   Big-headed person

increased risk for colon polyps and gastrointestinal polyps, which could eventually lead to colon cancer. Subjects with large head circumference were also seen to have increased risk of breast, uterine, and thyroid cancer (Fig. 1).

Dr. Sven Ove Samuelsen and colleagues have also steered a similar study at Public Health Institute, Norway where over a million health records of young people were examined over a long period of time. The researchers concluded: "We have found a strong and consistent positive relation between head circumference at birth and brain cancer in childhood." For every 1 cm increase in head circumference, a relative risk of 27% was shown. "To our knowledge, this is the first study to report an association between increased head circumference at birth and brain cancer in childhood," Dr. Samuelsen said. "Our findings suggest that brain pathology originates during foetal life in children diagnosed with brain cancer," he added.

These findings only reveal an association between cancer risk and head circumference and not cause and effect. This should not raise any alarm for people with big heads as further research is needed to firmly establish this link with molecular explanation to that effect. There is more to cancer development and head size cannot be the sole contributing factor. A possible explanation to this link has been attributed to hormones and growth factors. The growth of both healthy and tumor cells is driven by growth factors, hence there is a likelihood of influence from these factors. Another hypothesis also says that big heads contain more cells hence there is a high probability of cell division, mutation, and abnormal cell growth. People with increased head circumference can visit a genetic counselor to determine whether they should be screened for breast, uterine, colon, and thyroid cancers. These findings should be welcomed as it opens another dimension of cancer research to improve cancer diagnosis, treatment, and management.

Bibliography

Heald B, Mester J, Rybicki L, Orloff MS, Burke CA, Eng C. (2010). Frequent gastrointestinal polyps and colorectal adenocarcinomas in a prospective series of PTEN mutation carriers. *Gastroenterology, 139*(6), 1927–1933. doi:10.1053/j.gastro.2010.06.061.

Samuelsen SO, Bakketeig LS, Tretli S, Johannesen TB, Magnus P. (2006). Head circumference at birth and risk of brain cancer in childhood: A population-based study. *The Lancet Oncology, 7*(1), 39–42. doi:10.1016/S1470-2045(05)70470-8.

Tan MH, Mester J, Peterson C, *et al.* (2011). A clinical scoring system for selection of patients for PTEN mutation testing is proposed on the basis of a prospective study of 3042 probands. *American Journal of Human Genetics, 88*(1), 42–56. doi:10.1016/j.ajhg.2010.11.013.

Chapter 17

Increased Cancer Risk for Tall People

The spotlight has mostly been on weight anytime cancer is linked to a physical trait. This might be so because of the intensive studies that have been focused on this area of research. Another spectrum of research that has emerged recently is the association between height and cancer risk. People can easily trace meaning to weight and cancer association but would hardly believe the height/cancer link.

Studies have identified strong links between height and cancer risk. A study led by Geoffrey Kabat, Department of Epidemiology and Population Health, Albert Einstein College of Medicine and published in the journal *Cancer Epidemiology, Biomarkers and Prevention*, analyzed about 20,928 postmenopausal women and the factors that contribute to their health. The researchers discovered that per every 10 cm increase in height, there is a correlating 13% increased risk of developing a range of cancers at 19 sites including: rectum, thyroid, kidney, endometrium, colon, ovary, breast multiple myeloma, and malignant melanoma. A striking 23–29% increased risk was revealed for kidney, rectum, thyroid, and blood cancers (Fig. 1).

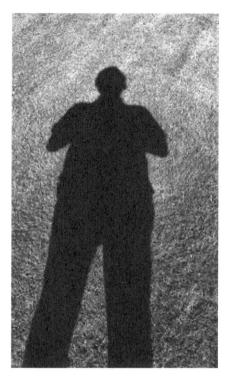

Fig. 1. A shadow of a tall person

In a large nested case-control study and meta-analysis conducted at the Department of Social Medicine, University of Bristol and published in *Cancer Epidemiology, Biomarkers and Prevention,* Luisa Zuccolo and colleagues established a significantly positive association between height and high-grade prostate cancer in British men. A similar trend has been shown in a prospective cohort study conducted by researchers from the University of Oxford and the Institut Catala d'Oncologia (ICO) in Barcelona and published in peer-reviewed medical journal *The Lancet Oncology.* In total 1.3 million participants were recruited in the United Kingdom with careful consideration of their alcohol intake, smoking habits, age, body mass index (BMI), weight, and other environmental factors that can possibly influence the outcome of the study. Six categories were created and the participants were placed into <155 cm, 155–159 cm, 160–164.9 cm, 165–169.9 cm, 170–174.9 cm, and ≥175 cm groups. Led by Dr. Jane Green, the researchers analyzed the height and cancer incidences of 17 sites including: mouth, throat, lung, pancreas, esophagus, stomach, ovary, colon, kidney, central nervous system, bladder, rectum, endometrium, blood cancers, and melanoma and also calculated the relative risk per 10 cm increase in height.

The findings of the study revealed that per 10 cm increase in height, there was a correlating 16% increased risk of developing any type of cancer considered. There was about 14–20% increased risk for rectal cancer, breast, endometrium, ovary, and central nervous system-related cancers. A striking 21–30% increased risk was shown for colon, malignant melanoma, kidney, non-Hodgkin's lymphoma, and leukemia. A similar height-associated risk was shown in a meta-analysis of this study and other 10 studies.

Despite the promising findings from this study, tall people should not be alarmed because this is just a connection, not a cause-and-effect association. Moreover, height alone cannot be singled out to be a cause of cancer development but rather a marker for something happening. The actual cause of this connection is not known as Dr. Green admitted: "The point is we don't know." However, scientists suggest growth factors like insulin-like growth factors and hormones drive the growth of height, likewise tumor cells. Another explanation is that taller people possess a greater number of cells and tissues hence provide a large surface area for cell division, mutation, and abnormal growth leading to tumor growth. Although height is mostly genetically dependent, environmental exposures or nutrition in early life could also affect the genes. For example, children born from 20 years ago to date have seen massive increase in height due to nutrition modification in the early stages of life. Also, people born in elite homes have a higher tendency of growing taller than those in the less elite setting. This is due to highly improved diets served in these highly educated homes.

Overall, there is overwhelming evidence suggesting possible associations between height and increased cancer risk as well as certain genetic mutations that predispose a person to cancer. These cancers include ovarian, colon, endometrial, breast, lung, and prostate cancers. However, mechanistic evidence is needed to warrant further clinical studies. These findings raise so many biological questions about the connection and the exact role of height in cancer development. This could stir up another area of research where researchers can identify and evaluate the mechanisms of growth factors and hormones that influence height and tumor growth at the same time. Once the molecular mechanisms underpinning the height/cancer association are unveiled, a more defined and well-tailored knowledge/explanation could be developed and treatment modalities affected as well. This is an interesting finding; however, much effort is needed to substantiate the link.

Bibliography

Bertrand KA, Gerlovin H, Bethea TN, Palmer JR. (2017). Pubertal growth and adult height in relation to breast cancer risk in African American women. *International Journal of Cancer, 141*(12), 2462–2470. doi:10.1002/ijc.31019.

Green J, Cairns BJ, Casabonne D, *et al.* (2011). Height and cancer incidence in the Million Women Study: Prospective cohort, and meta-analysis of prospective studies of height and total cancer risk. *The Lancet Oncology, 12*(8), 785–794. doi:10.1016/S1470-2045(11)70154-1.

Jing Z, Hou X, Liu Y, *et al.* (2015). Association between height and thyroid cancer risk: A meta-analysis of prospective cohort studies. *International Journal of Cancer, 137*(6), 1484–1490. doi:10.1002/ijc.29487.

Kabat GC, Heo M, Kamensky V, Miller AB, Rohan TE. (2013). Adult height in relation to risk of cancer in a cohort of Canadian women. *International Journal of Cancer, 132*(5), 1125–1132. Published online 2012, August 6. doi:10.1002/ijc.27704.

Khankari NK, Shu XO, Wen W, *et al.* (2016). Association between adult height and risk of colorectal, lung, and prostate cancer: Results from meta-analyses of prospective studies and Mendelian randomization analyses. *PLoS Medicine, 13*(9), e1002118. doi:10.1371/journal.pmed.1002118.

Kim SJ, Huzarski T, Gronwald J, *et al.* (2018). Prospective evaluation of body size and breast cancer risk among BRCA1 and BRCA2 mutation carriers. *International Journal of Epidemiology, 47*(3), 987–997. Advance online publication. doi:10.1093/ije/dyy039.

Lophatananon A, Stewart-Brown S, Kote-Jarai Z, *et al.* (2017). Height, selected genetic markers and prostate cancer risk: Results from the PRACTICAL consortium. *British Journal of Cancer, 117*(5), 734–743. doi:10.1038/bjc.2017.231.

Qian F, Rookus MA, Leslie G, *et al.* (2019). Mendelian randomisation study of height and body mass index as modifiers of ovarian cancer risk in 22,588 *BRCA1* and *BRCA2* mutation carriers. *British Journal of Cancer, 121*, 180–192. doi:10.1038/s41416-019-0492-8.

Thrift AP, Gong J, Peters U, *et al.* (2015). Mendelian randomization study of height and risk of colorectal cancer. *International Journal of Epidemiology, 44*(2), 662–672. doi:10.1093/ije/dyv082.

Wiedmann MKH, Brunborg C, Di Ieva A, *et al.* (2017). Overweight, obesity and height as risk factors for meningioma, glioma, pituitary adenoma and nerve sheath tumor: A large population-based prospective cohort study. *Acta Oncologica, 56*(10), 1302–1309. doi:10.1080/0284186X.2017.1330554.

Wirén S, Häggström C, Ulmer H, *et al.* (2014). Pooled cohort study on height and risk of cancer and cancer death. *Cancer Causes & Control: CCC, 25*(2), 151–159. doi:10.1007/s10552-013-0317-7.

Zhang B, Shu XO, Delahanty RJ, *et al.* (2015). Height and breast cancer risk: Evidence from prospective studies and Mendelian randomization. *Journal of the National Cancer Institute, 107*(11), djv219. doi:10.1093/jnci/djv219.

Zuccolo L, Harris R, Gunnell D, *et al.* (2008). Height and prostate cancer risk: A large nested case-control study (ProtecT) and meta-analysis. *Cancer Epidemiology, Biomarkers & Prevention: A Publication of the American Association for Cancer Research, Cosponsored by the American Society of Preventive Oncology, 17*(9), 2325–2336. doi:10.1158/1055-9965.EPI-08-0342.

Chapter 18

Do Snorers Have Increased Risk of Cancer Death?

Sleep is a natural part of the life of humans and other living organisms where the individual has a reduced perception of environmental stimuli. This is a state where the body is put into a mood of relaxation and rejuvenation. Despite sleep being of a total health benefit, there are disorders that are related to sleep and can interfere with mental, social, spiritual, physical, and emotional well-being. Sleeping disorder or somnipathy could be broadly categorized under dyssomnias, parasomnias, circadian rhythm sleep disorders, and medical-related sleeping disorders.

It's not only annoying and irritating sleeping next to a person who snores; you are also sleeping close to someone who has increased risk of cancer death. I know it's quite surprising to know that snoring and sleep-disordered breathing (SDB) have been linked to increased risk of cancer deaths. A well-controlled cohort study conducted by a group of scientists from the University of Wisconsin and University of Barcelona has revealed a link between SDB — includes snoring — and cancer death (Fig. 1).

The 22-year study recruited 1,522 adults with a well-monitored sleep at a sleep laboratory. Based on a standardized "apnea–hypo-

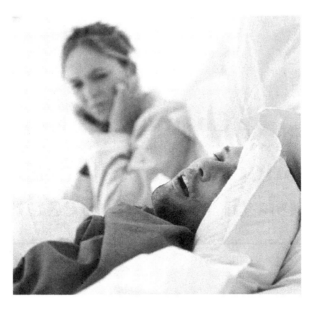

Fig. 1. A snorer

pnea index" (AHI) scale, the subjects were categorized as normal sleep breathing, mild SDB, moderate SDB, and severe SDB based on their score. The researchers also took into consideration other parameters that can affect the risk of cancer such as age, gender, smoking habits, alcohol consumption, physical activity, other medical records — diabetes and sleeping apnea — and body mass index (BMI).

Among the recruited participants, 24% (365) of them had SDB with the following divisions: 14.6% considered as mild, 5.5% as moderate, and 3.9% as severe. People in the worst SDB division were reported to also have increased BMIs, predominantly males, less educated, and with poor health status. During the follow-up exercise, 50 cancer-related deaths were recorded and represented as 3.2% of the mild SDB group, 6% of the moderate SDB group, 11.9% of the severe SDB group, and 2.7% of the normal sleep breathing group. The researchers reported that, people with severe SDB are 4.8 times more likely to die from cancer than people with normal sleeping breathing. The results generated from the mild and moderate groups were not significant enough to be linked to cancer death.

Laboratory and animal experiments have earlier revealed that low oxygen levels in mice promote and favor tumor growth by angiogenesis — a process where new blood vessels are generated in order to support tumor cells. Scientists therefore believe the low oxygen levels identified in some snorers or people with SDB may drive tumor growth, hence stopping snoring could be of therapeutic benefit to cancer patients. "The consistency of the evidence from the animal experiments and this new epidemiologic evidence in humans is highly compelling," Dr. Javier Nieto, the leader of the study noted. Nevertheless, this is the first study to point out an association between snoring/SDB and increased cancer mortality. Further studies are therefore needed to establish and prove this link or association.

This study presents an interesting finding that must be commended. However, there are some caveats that need to be addressed to improve further studies. The number of SDB subjects was small hence the number of deaths recorded in that was also small. There is a high probability that this small figure could be influenced by chance or other factors. A larger study is recommended to give a through reflection of the link. Despite taking into consideration other factors that can affect the results like alcohol consumption, BMI, and others, there is a probability that the findings might have been affected by some unmentioned factors as well. This study is mainly about the risk of cancer death but not the risk of getting cancer. It will be more advantageous if the latter is also considered in future research. After future cohort studies have firmly established the association between snoring and SDB and cancer risk/death, the animal studies should be replicated in humans to gather enough molecular and cellular evidence to buttress the link. Other studies have also shown significant correlation between SDB and lung cancer risk. This being the first study to reveal such association, there should be more studies to confirm the link. Notwithstanding, the findings are interesting and should spark another field of research into other sleeping disorders.

It is very interesting to note that sleep difficulty also affects the immune system especially tumor-fighting immune cells. In a study published in the *Sleep* journal, natural killer cells were reported to be very low. This phenomenon was associated with increased risk of cancer. As to whether the sleep condition resulted in the decreased immune cells or vice versa is yet to be investigated. When this link is firmly established, targeting sleeping disorders like SDB could possibly increase the survival of cancer patients.

Bibliography

Christensen AS, Clark A, Salo P, *et al.* (2013). Symptoms of sleep disordered breathing and risk of cancer: A prospective cohort study. *Sleep, 36*(10), 1429–1435. doi:10.5665/sleep.3030.

Daniel LC, Wang M, Mulrooney DA, *et al.* (2019). Sleep, emotional distress, and physical health in survivors of childhood cancer: A report from the childhood cancer survivor study. *Psychooncology, 28*(4), 903–912. doi:10.1002/pon.5040.

Dreher M, Krüger S, Schulze-Olden S, *et al.* (2018). Sleep-disordered breathing in patients with newly diagnosed lung cancer. *BMC Pulmonary Medicine, 18*, 72. doi:10.1186/s12890-018-0645-1.

Gaoatswe G, Kent BD, Corrigan MA, *et al.* (2015). Invariant natural killer T cell deficiency and functional impairment in sleep apnea: Links to cancer comorbidity. *Sleep, 38*(10), 1629–1634. doi:10.5665/sleep.5062.

Liu W, Luo M, Fang Y, *et al.* (2019). Relationship between occurrence and progression of lung cancer and nocturnal intermittent hypoxia, apnea and daytime sleepiness. *Current Medical Science, 39*, 568. doi:10.1007/s11596-019-2075-6.

Nieto FJ, Peppard PE, Young T, Finn L, Hla KM, Farré R. (2012). Sleep-disordered breathing and cancer mortality: Results from the Wisconsin Sleep Cohort Study. *American Journal of Respiratory and Critical Care Medicine, 186*(2), 190–194. doi:10.1164/rccm.201201-0130OC.

Pérez-Warnisher MT, Fernanda Troncoso M, Cabezas E, *et al.* (2017). Sleep disordered breathing is very prevalent in patients with lung cancer: Preliminary results of the SAIL study (Sleep Apnea In Lung cancer). *European Respiratory Journal, 50*(Suppl.61),PA4241.doi:10.1183/1393003. congress-2017.PA4241.

Phipps AI, Bhatti P, Neuhouser ML, *et al.* (2016). Pre-diagnostic sleep duration and sleep quality in relation to subsequent cancer survival. *Journal* of *Clinical Sleep Medicine: JCSM: Official Publication of the American Academy of Sleep Medicine, 12*(4), 495–503. doi:10.5664/jcsm.5674.

Zhang X, Giovannucci EL, Wu K, *et al.* (2013). Associations of self-reported sleep duration and snoring with colorectal cancer risk in men and women. *Sleep, 36*(5), 681–688. doi:10.5665/sleep.2626.

Chapter 19

Dogs: The New Era of "Oncologists"

Being nicknamed as "man's best friend," domestic dogs are considered to be one of the friendliest animals to humans. With an estimation of about 700 million to over 1 billion dogs in the world, the origin of this group of canivora is still not clearly known. They serve many useful and unique purposes in most parts of the world such as hunting, companionship, police assistance, aide for the disabled, sports, and protection. In the developed world, domestic dogs are seen as integral members of the family with some couples substituting their kids for them. However, in some parts of Asia — South Korea, China, and Vietnam — and Africa, dogs are purposely raised for their meat. This might sound awkward to those who consider dogs as "family members."

Domestic dogs also present a major health risk to humans; 1.8% of American population is bitten by dogs each year with other dog-related murder cases being reported in some parts of the world. Toxocariasis, where a human is infected with roundworm eggs from dog feces, has also been detected in a significant number of the populace in both America and United Kingdom. Notwithstanding, the medical importance of dogs cannot be underestimated. Psychological, physical, and social well-being have been shown to be enhanced through companionship with dogs. The latest discovery is the incredible association between domestically trained dogs and cancer detection.

Cancer continues to claim lives and has comfortably earned the accolade as one of the deadliest diseases. With more than a million deaths recorded worldwide each year, there is the urgent need for a more accurate and efficient diagnosis even in the early stages. It is in this regard that research scientists have discovered novel and state-of-the-art techniques for detecting cancer using body fluids and other specimens. Such groundbreaking approaches could contribute to early detection and treatment as well as increase survival rate. Cancer scientists have done the unbelievable by exploring the olfactory system in dogs to detect cancer-related compounds through the sniffing of body fluids such as urine. Substantial amount of data has been reported detailing the prospects of using highly trained animals especially dogs to detect cancer (Fig. 1).

In 2006, Michael McCulloch and colleagues of San Anselmo, California, embarked on a study where five ordinary trained house dogs were used to detect both lung and breast cancers by sniffing breath samples. In total 55 lung cancer and 31 breast cancer samples

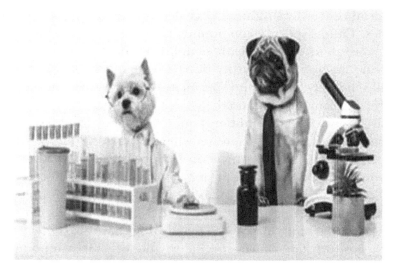

Fig. 1. Dogs working at the lab

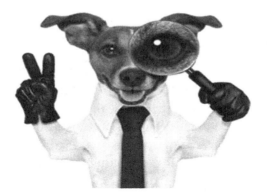

Fig. 2.   A dog researcher

were used in the experiment together with 83 healthy control samples. The overall sensitivity for lung cancer detection was 99%, likewise the overall specificity. The overall sensitivity and specificity for breast cancer detection were recorded as 88% and 98%, respectively (Fig. 2).

A similar research was conducted at the Department of Surgery and Science, Kyushu University, Japan by Dr. Hideto Sonoda, where one specially trained dog — Labrador retriever — was used to detect colorectal cancer by sniffing 33 exhaled breath and 37 watery stool samples. Cancer-specific compounds resulting in a specific cancer scent were detected in breath samples by the Labrador retriever, achieving an overall sensitivity of 91% and specificity of 99%. An overall sensitivity of 97% and specificity of 99% were achieved when watery stool samples were used.

BBC News Health Editor, James Gallagher in March 2015 reported a study by US scientists where Frankie, a highly trained dog, sniffed out thyroid cancer in people who had not yet been diagnosed. Frankie had 30 out of 34 urine samples correct, achieving 88% success rate. These amazing findings have been presented at the annual meeting of the Endocrine Society.

Two highly trained 3-year-old female dogs have also detected the presence of prostate cancer-specific volatile organic compounds in urine samples with more than 90% accuracy. Gianluigi Taverna and colleagues in Milan recruited 362 prostate cancer patients and 540 healthy control samples to achieve such an amazing finding. This incredible result has also been featured in the April 2015 news of *The Guardian* and NHS UK. This evolving technique presents an incredible means of substituting the invasive procedure of diagnosing some of these cancers and comes as good news for patients who are not fond of the needle. In addition to that, this procedure could be highly patronized and useful in areas where biopsy is difficult to access.

These findings reported are based on the extraordinary and unique structure of the olfactory system in dogs. Their olfactory bulb is about 40 times bigger than that of humans, with 125–220 million smell-sensitive receptors. Thus, dogs generally possess a very high sense-sensitivity, hence their incredible scent detection.

Despite the promising sniffing technique exhibited by these dogs, their clinical use is a bit questionable. The widespread use of dogs will not be ideal especially with problems of accuracy. It is therefore prudent to detect the cancer-related chemicals or compounds that are perceived by the olfactory system of the dogs. By so doing, the use of dogs in the lab would be prevented while accuracy is maximized and well controlled under standardized procedures. Dr. Emma Smith of Cancer Research UK has suggested the need for electronic nose that could be more practicable to be used in the laboratories to detect the same molecules or chemicals detected by these trained dogs.

This opens another research field to explore the olfactory systems of other animals to detect cancer-related molecules. Beside dogs, other animals like guinea pigs, horses, rats, elephants, and mice have also been reported to have a very high amount of smell receptors. Future discoveries in such animals will add up to the proposed e-nose diagnosing technique, leading to more specific e-nose for specific cancers. Who knows if the sensory receptors of any of those animals will be more specific for some particular cancers? One likely challenge to be encountered is the training of these animals to detect unique scent relating to cancer. A close examination of the various breeds of dogs to identify the group that possesses more sensitivity to smell will also be useful. This will further direct a new field to engineer dogs with very high smell sensitivity.

Cells from different types of cancer have unique odors that could be identified by trained dogs. Using these odor differences, trained dogs employ their strong olfactory system to detect colorectal cancers with a sensitivity and specificity of 91% and 99%, respectively. Odors from patients in early stages of cancer were highly detected compared with late stages. Using patient breath, trained dogs were able to detect patients with liver cancers. In a separate study, blood serum was used to diagnose patients with non-small cell lung cancer.

With the quest to help disarm cancer worldwide, this promising technique is highly welcomed. However, there is more to be done to make this practicable in the clinics. Cancer research scientists are forever determined to pursue the course of championing the war against the deadly canker, cancer.

Bibliography

Biehl W, Hattesohl A, Jörres RA, *et al.* (2019). VOC pattern recognition of lung cancer: A comparative evaluation of different dog- and eNose-based strategies using different sampling materials. *Acta Oncologica, 58,* 1216–1224. doi:10.1080/0284186X.2019.1634284.

de Boer NK, de Meij TG, Oort FA, *et al.* (2014). The scent of colorectal cancer: Detection by volatile organic compound analysis. *Clinical Gastroenterology and Hepatology: The Official Clinical Practice Journal of the American Gastroenterological Association, 12*(7), 1085–1089. doi:10.1016/j.cgh.2014.05.005.

Dorman DC, Foster ML, Fernhoff KE, Hess PR. (2017). Canine scent detection of canine cancer: A feasibility study. *Veterinary Medicine (Auckland, N.Z.), 8,* 69–76. doi:10.2147/VMRR.S148594.

Ehmann R, Boedeker E, Friedrichet U, *et al.* (2012). Canine scent detection in the diagnosis of lung cancer: Revisiting a puzzling phenomenon. *European Respiratory Journal, 39*(3), 669–676. doi:10.1183/09031936.00051711.

The Endocrine Society. (2015, March 7). Scent-trained dog detects thyroid cancer in human urine samples. *ScienceDaily.* Retrieved October 26, 2019 from www.sciencedaily.com/releases/2015/03/150307095943.htm.

Gordon RT, Schatz CB, Myers LJ, *et al.* (2008). The use of canines in the detection of human cancers. *The Journal of Alternative and Complementary Medicine: Research on Paradigm, Practice, and Policy, 14*(1), 61–67. doi:10.1089/acm.2006.6408.

Hackner K, Errhalt P, Mueller MR, *et al.* (2016). Canine scent detection for the diagnosis of lung cancer in a screening-like situation. *Journal of Breath Research, 10,* 046003.

Horvath G, Järverud GA, Järverud S, Horváth I. (2008). Human ovarian carcinomas detected by specific odor. *Integrative Cancer Therapies, 7,* 76–80. doi:10.1177/1534735408319058.

Junqueira H, Quinn TA, Biringer R, *et al.* (2019). Accuracy of canine scent detection of non–small cell lung cancer in blood serum. *The Journal of the American Osteopathic Association, 119*(7), 413–418. doi:10.7556/jaoa. 2019.077.

Kitiyakara T, Redmond S, Unwanatham N, *et al.* (2017). The detection of hepatocellular carcinoma (HCC) from patients' breath using canine scent detection: A proof-of-concept study. *Journal of Breath Research, 11,* 046002.

McCulloch M, Jezierski T, Broffman M, Hubbard A, Turner K, Janecki T. (2006). Diagnostic accuracy of canine scent detection in early- and late-stage lung and breast cancers. *Integrative Cancer Therapies, 5*(1), 30–39. doi:10.1177/1534735405285096.

Sonoda H, Kohnoe S, Yamazato T, *et al.* (2011). Colorectal cancer screening with odour material by canine scent detection. *Gut, 60*(6), 814–819. doi:10.1136/gut.2010.218305.

Taverna G, Tidu L, Grizzi F, *et al.* (2015). Olfactory system of highly trained dogs detects prostate cancer in urine samples. *The Journal of Urology, 193*(4), 1382–1387. doi:10.1016/j.juro.2014.09.099.

Chapter 20

Is Cannabis (CBD) an Alternative Cancer Treatment Agent?

Cannabis is derived from the cannabis plant and contains several bioactive agents known collectively as cannabinoids. There is one of the cannabinoids, THC (delta-9-tetrahydrocannabinol), which has been shown to possess psychoactive properties known to cause hallucinations, mental confusion, and drowsiness. Unlike THC, cannabidiol (CBD) doesn't possess any psychoactive properties and has been shown to offer protection against several disease conditions (Fig. 1). There are many people who use cannabis for recreational purposes and depending on the geographical location, this might be considered legal or not. In Canada, recreational use of cannabis is legal and regularized by the Canadian government.

Excessive cannabis use could lead to serious health implications such as cognitive impairment, chronic bronchitis, lung inflammation, fetal damage in pregnant women as well as nervous breakdown. Reports indicate that rare forms of cancer have been reported in women who took higher dose of cannabis during pregnancy. To date, cannabis is banned in about 98% of countries in the world and

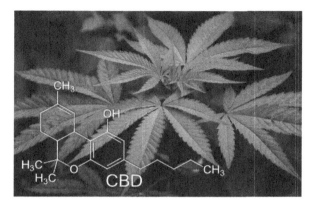

Fig. 1. Cannabis plant and a CBD chemical formula

it's therefore illegal to use it regardless of the intended purpose. Regardless of the controversies surrounding cannabis, recent evidence demonstrates its therapeutic properties in a plethora of diseases such as schizophrenia, chronic inflammation and pain, asthma, glaucoma, nausea, and vomiting associated with advanced chronic diseases.

Extracts from cannabis have shown promise as anticancer protection or prevention agents especially CBD. Receptors that receive signals from cannabinoids are highly expressed on various tumor tissues and hence respond to the treatment of cannabinoids. CBD has been demonstrated to suppress tumor-promoting signals, reduce tumor growth, and inhibit angiogenesis and metastasis. CBD also promotes programmed cell death in cancer cells and leads to the reduction of cancer cell growth. This has been shown in breast, ovarian, lung, prostate, melanoma, endometrial, colorectal, and head-and-neck cancer cell lines. The legal regulations surrounding cannabis usage have in a way impeded the research progress compared with bioactive agents from other plants. This is in part due to insufficient funding agencies willing to support cannabis research. Religious beliefs also play a huge role in slowing down the usage of cannabis for therapeutic purposes. Most religious bodies demonize cannabis plants and thus, do not encourage members to explore their therapeutic properties regardless of how effective they will be.

Lack of education has also contributed to the slow cannabis research in that, most people have the mindset that nothing good comes out of cannabis and their main and only function is their psychoactive effect. This is entirely not true since only one of the cannabinoids (THC) is related to the psychoactive effect of the plant.

Due to the lack of highly robust laboratories that can fractionize and separate the various cannabinoids, most people use the entire cannabis plant and therefore end up with cognitive impairments. Another way to promote the medical usage of cannabis is to genetically engineer cannabis to produce no THC but high amount of medically relevant cannabinoids such as CBD. This will minimize the abuse of cannabis for their psychoactive properties but rather channel more efforts into their research.

Currently, there are two chemically synthesized drugs based on the formulation of cannabis that have been approved by FDA to be used in the United States:

1. Dronabinol (Marinol®) contains THC that has been approved to treat nausea and vomiting caused by chemotherapeutic treatments in cancer patients. This drug has proven to be helpful in AIDS patients suffering from weight loss and loss of appetite.
2. Nabilone (Cesamet®) is a synthetic compound formulated in the likeness of THC. It also works like dronabinol and is highly used in chemotherapeutic treatments to alleviate nausea and vomiting.

In the United States, Nabiximols is being tested in the clinics as a mouth spray with a composition of both THC and CBD in equal amounts. Although currently not approved by the FDA, Nabiximol is available in the United States, Canada, and some parts of Europe and indicated for the treatment of cancer-related pains, muscle spasms, and the management of multiple sclerosis (MS).

Although cannabis has shown promise in cancer prevention and treatment, further mechanistic studies are required to substantiate these findings. This will provide solid rationale for these bioactive agents to be tested in the clinics and approved by the FDA. Researchers could also explore the possibility of combining FDA-approved cancer drugs with cannabinoids to see if patients' survival will be much improved compared with single treatments. The abuse of cannabis is detrimental to the health; however, their medical properties could be exploited to enhance patients' survival.

Bibliography

Andre CM, Hausman JF, Guerriero G. (2016). *Cannabis sativa*: The plant of the thousand and one molecules. *Frontiers in Plant Science, 7,* 19. doi:10.3389/fpls.2016.00019.

Caffarel MM, Andradas C, Mira E, *et al.* (2010). Cannabinoids reduce ErbB2-driven breast cancer progression through Akt inhibition. *Molecular Cancer, 9,* 196. doi:10.1186/1476-4598-9-196.

Caffarel MM, Andradas C, Perez-Gomez E, Guzman M, Sanchez C. (2012). Cannabinoids: A new hope for breast cancer therapy? *Cancer Treatment Reviews, 38*(7), 911–918. doi:10.1016/j.ctrv.2012.06.005.

Carracedo A, Gironella M, Lorente M, *et al.* (2006). Cannabinoids induce apoptosis of pancreatic tumor cells via endoplasmic reticulum stress-related genes. *Cancer Research, 66*(13), 6748–6755. doi:10.1158/0008-5472.CAN-06-0169.

Chakravarti B, Ravi J, Ganju RK. (2014). Cannabinoids as therapeutic agents in cancer: Current status and future implications. *Oncotarget, 5*(15), 5852–5872. doi:10.18632/oncotarget.2233.

Chung SC, Hammarsten P, Josefsson A, *et al.* (2009). A high cannabinoid CB1 receptor immunoreactivity is associated with disease severity and outcome in prostate cancer. *European Journal of Cancer, 45*(1), 174–182. doi:10.1016/j.ejca.2008.10.010.

Cipriano M, Haggstrom J, Hammarsten P, Fowler CJ. (2013). Association between cannabinoid CB1 receptor expression and Akt signalling in prostate cancer. *PLoS One, 8*(6), e65798. doi:10.1371/journal.pone.0065798.

De Petrocellis L, Ligresti A, Moriello AS, *et al.* (2011). Effects of cannabinoids and cannabinoid-enriched Cannabis extracts on TRP channels and endocannabinoid metabolic enzymes. *British Journal of Pharmacology, 163*(7), 1479–1494. doi:10.1111/j.1476-5381.2010.01166.x.

De Petrocellis L, Ligresti A, Moriello AS, *et al.* (2013). Non-THC cannabinoids inhibit prostate carcinoma growth in vitro and in vivo: Pro-apoptotic effects and underlying mechanisms. *British Journal of Pharmacology, 168*(1), 79–102. doi:10.1111/j.1476-5381.2012.02027.x.

Demuth DG, Molleman A. (2006). Cannabinoid signalling. *Life Sciences,* *78*(6), 549–563. doi:10.1016/j.lfs.2005.05.055.

Fogli S, Nieri P, Chicca A, *et al.* (2006). Cannabinoid derivatives induce cell death in pancreatic MIA PaCa-2 cells via a receptor-independent mechanism. *FEBS Letters, 580*(7), 1733–1739. doi:10.1016/j.febslet. 2006.02.024.

Freund P, Porpaczy EA, Le T, *et al.* (2016). Cannabinoid receptors are overexpressed in CLL but of limited potential for therapeutic exploitation. *PLoS One, 11*(6), e0156693. doi:10.1371/journal.pone.0156693.

Guzman M. (2003). Cannabinoids: Potential anticancer agents. *Nature Reviews Cancer, 3*(10), 745–755. doi:10.1038/nrc1188.

Malfitano AM, Ciaglia E, Gangemi G, Gazzerro P, Laezza C, Bifulco M. (2011). Update on the endocannabinoid system as an anticancer target. *Expert Opinion on Therapeutic Targets, 15*(3), 297–308. doi:10.1517/ 14728222.2011.553606.

Michalski CW, Oti FE, Erkan M, *et al.* (2008). Cannabinoids in pancreatic cancer: Correlation with survival and pain. *International Journal of Cancer, 122*(4), 742–750. doi:10.1002/ijc.23114.

Mukhopadhyay B, Schuebel K, Mukhopadhyay P, *et al.* (2015). Cannabinoid receptor 1 promotes hepatocellular carcinoma initiation and progression through multiple mechanisms. *Hepatology, 61*(5), 1615–1626. doi:10.1002/hep.27686.

Nomura DK, Long JZ, Niessen S, Hoover HS, Ng SW, Cravatt BF. (2010). Monoacylglycerol lipase regulates a fatty acid network that promotes cancer pathogenesis. *Cell, 140*(1), 49–61. doi:10.1016/j.cell.2009.11.027.

Orellana-Serradell O, Poblete CE, Sanchez C, *et al.* (2015). Proapoptotic effect of endocannabinoids in prostate cancer cells. *Oncology Reports, 33*(4), 1599–1608. doi:10.3892/or.2015.3746.

Pecze L, Josvay K, Blum W, *et al.* (2016). Activation of endogenous TRPV1 fails to induce overstimulation-based cytotoxicity in breast and prostate cancer cells but not in pain-sensing neurons. *Biochimica et Biophysica Acta, 1863*(8), 2054–2064. doi:10.1016/j.bbamcr.2016.05.007.

Perez-Gomez E, Andradas C, Blasco-Benito S, *et al.* (2015). Role of cannabinoid receptor CB2 in HER2 pro-oncogenic signaling in breast cancer. *Journal of the National Cancer Institute, 107*(6), djv077. doi:10.1093/jnci/ djv077.

Pineiro R, Maffucci T, Falasca M. (2011). The putative cannabinoid receptor GPR55 defines a novel autocrine loop in cancer cell proliferation. *Oncogene, 30*(2), 142–152. doi:10.1038/onc.2010.417.

Preet A, Qamri Z, Nasser MW, *et al.* (2011). Cannabinoid receptors, CB1 and CB2, as novel targets for inhibition of non-small cell lung cancer growth and metastasis. *Cancer Prevention Research (Philadelphia, PA.)*, *4*(1), 65–75. doi:10.1158/1940-6207.CAPR-10-0181.

Romano B, Pagano E, Orlando P, *et al.* (2016). Pure delta9-tetrahydrocannabivarin and a *Cannabis sativa* extract with high content in delta9-tetrahydrocannabivarin inhibit nitrite production in murine peritoneal macrophages. *Pharmacological Research, 113*(Pt A), 199–208. doi:10.1016/j.phrs.2016.07.045.

Sanchez MG, Sanchez AM, Collado B, *et al.* (2005). Expression of the transient receptor potential vanilloid 1 (TRPV1) in LNCaP and PC-3 prostate cancer cells and in human prostate tissue. *European Journal of Pharmacology, 515*(1–3), 20–27. doi:10.1016/j.ejphar.2005.04.010.

Sarfaraz S, Adhami VM, Syed DN, Afaq F, Mukhtar H. (2008). Cannabinoids for cancer treatment: Progress and promise. *Cancer Research, 68*(2), 339–342. doi:10.1158/0008-5472.CAN-07-2785.

Thors L, Bergh A, Persson E, *et al.* (2010). Fatty acid amide hydrolase in prostate cancer: Association with disease severity and outcome, CB1 receptor expression and regulation by IL-4. *PLoS One, 5*(8), e12275. doi:10.1371/journal.pone.0012275.

Velasco G, Hernandez S, Davila D, Lorente M. (2016). The use of cannabinoids as anticancer agents. *Progress in Neuro-Psychopharmacology & Biological Psychiatry, 64*, 259–266. doi:10.1016/j.pnpbp.2015.05.010.

Velasco G, Sanchez C, Guzman M. (2015). Endocannabinoids and cancer. *Handbook of Experimental Pharmacology, 231*, 449–472. doi:10.1007/978-3-319-20825-1_16.

Velasco G, Sanchez C, Guzman M. (2016). Anticancer mechanisms of cannabinoids. *Current Oncology, 23*(Suppl. 2), S23–S32. doi:10.3747/co.23.3080.

Vercelli C, Barbero R, Cuniberti B, *et al.* (2014). Transient receptor potential vanilloid 1 expression and functionality in MCF-7 cells: A preliminary investigation. *Journal of Breast Cancer, 17*(4), 332–338. doi:10.4048/jbc.2014.17.4.332.

Xu X, Liu Y, Huang S, *et al.* (2006). Overexpression of cannabinoid receptors CB1 and CB2 correlates with improved prognosis of patients with hepatocellular carcinoma. *Cancer Genetics and Cytogenetics, 171*(1), 31–38. doi:10.1016/j.cancergencyto.2006.06.014.

Zhao Z, Yang J, Zhao H, Fang X, Li H. (2012). Cannabinoid receptor 2 is upregulated in melanoma. *Journal of Cancer Research and Therapeutics, 8*(4), 549–554. doi:10.4103/0973-1482.106534.

Chapter 21

Vaping: An Emerging Concern for Increased Cancer Risk

E-cigarette smoking, popularly known as vaping, has been in the news of late but definitely not for the good reasons. E-cigarette is a battery-powered handheld electronic device that provides a similar feeling as smoking but without tobacco. E-cig, however, might contain nicotine and other products such as glycerol, glycol, and fruit flavors. The contents are in the form of juice that is heated and inhaled. Vaping is mostly seen as a less harmful means of cigarette smoking, which is not entirely true. This has attracted most young and old people to be involved in vaping thinking the harm being caused is minimal (Fig. 1).

Recent studies have shown that vaping has serious consequences on the users and could result in increased cancer risk. In a study published in the *International Journal of Molecular Sciences*, significant important genes were dysregulated in vapers and these dysregulations were similar to those in cigarette smokers. This is a huge public health concern that calls for instant regulation of e-cigarettes and tobacco-related products.

In another study published in *PNAS*, researchers at the New York University exposed 45 laboratory mice to nicotine-containing vapor, 4 hours a day for 5 days a week, over a 54-week period. The other

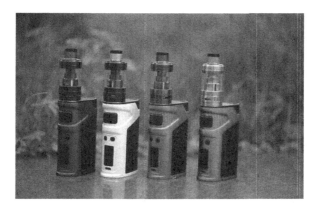

Fig. 1. Different flavors of e-cigarette on display

cohort of mice was either exposed to nicotine-free vapor or filtered air from the laboratory. Lung tumors were observed in 23% of the mice that were exposed to nicotine-laced vapor compared with the other groups. In this same group, 58% of the mice developed bladder urothelial hyperplasia, lesions that have high probability of turning into cancer.

There were, however, limitations in the study as a small number of mice were used in the study. Also, the rate and amount of vapor inhaled by the mice compared with humans might be different. Another limitation is that mice cannot inhale as deeply as humans, meaning more damage could result if vaping continues for a long while and the changes could even be worse. The vaping community sees this research as a means of fighting against the vaping industry and hence pays no regard to such studies. Narcotic regulatory bodies have also reported a rare form of lung disease outbreak that is related to vaping. There have been several reports that most of the e-cigarettes contain harmful constituents contrary to what is advertised and as a result pose a serious health threat to users. Pro-vaping groups have disregarded these findings, claiming the mice were allegedly exposed to larger quantities of nicotine-laced vapor that is unrealistic in humans.

In another related study, nicotine-laced vapor and its metabolites caused damage to DNA repair genes. This resulted in the development of lung and bladder cancers as well as complicated health conditions. E-cigarette-mediated DNA damage has also been reported in another study published in *Scientific Reports*. These results are alarming and should be taken seriously since the association between vaping and cancer risk has been proven at the cellular, preclinical, and clinical levels. Thinking that vaping is a less harmful means to smoke might be deceitful and cause lots of health damage. Vaping's association with cancer is regardless of race, sex, and lifestyle. Thus, the constituents of the e-cigarettes should be critically looked at. Help should be sought from experts when quitting smoking and vaping should not be used as an alternative.

Bibliography

Canistro D, Vivarelli F, Cirillo S, *et al.* (2017). E-cigarettes induce toxicological effects that can raise the cancer risk. *Scientific Reports, 7*(1), 2028. doi:10.1038/s41598-017-02317-8.

Fuller TW, Acharya AP, Meyyappan T, *et al.* (2018). Comparison of bladder carcinogens in the urine of e-cigarette users versus non e-cigarette using controls. *Scientific Reports, 8*(1), 507. doi:10.1038/s41598-017-19030-1.

Hajek P, Phillips-Waller A, Przulj D, *et al.* (2019). A randomized trial of e-cigarettes versus nicotine-replacement therapy. *The New England Journal of Medicine, 380*, 629–637. doi:10.1056/NEJMoa1808779.

Harris CC. (2018). Tobacco smoking, E-cigarettes, and nicotine harm. *Proceedings of the National Academy of Sciences, 115*(7), 1406–1407. doi:10.1073/pnas.1722636115.

Lee HW, Park S-H, Weng M-W, *et al.* (2018). E-cig damages DNA in lung, heart, and bladder. *Proceedings of the National Academy of Sciences, USA, 115*(7), E1560–E1569. doi:10.1073/pnas.1718185115.

Mravec B, Tibensky M, Horvathova L, Babal P. (2019, October 16). E-cigarettes and cancer risk. *Cancer Prevention Research.* doi:10.1158/1940-6207.CAPR-19-0346.

Rhoades DA, Comiford AL, Dvorak JD, *et al.* (2019). Vaping patterns, nicotine dependence and reasons for vaping among American Indian dual users of cigarettes and electronic cigarettes. *BMC Public Health, 19*(1), 1211. doi:10.1186/s12889-019-7523-5.

Schier JG, Meiman JG, Layden J, *et al.* (2019). Severe pulmonary disease associated with electronic-cigarette-product use — Interim guidance. *MMWR. Morbidity and Mortality Weekly Report, 68*(36), 787–790. doi: 10.15585/mmwr.mm6836e2.

Schuller HM. (2019). The impact of smoking and the influence of other factors on lung cancer, *Expert Review of Respiratory Medicine, 13*(8), 761–769. doi:10.1080/17476348.2019.1645010.

Son Y, Wackowski O, Weisel C, *et al.* (2018). Evaluation of e-vapor nicotine and nicotyrine concentrations under various e-liquid compositions, device settings, and vaping topographies. *Chemical Research in Toxicology, 31*(9), 861–868. doi:10.1021/acs.chemrestox.8b00063.

Stephens WE. (2018). Comparing the cancer potencies of emissions from vapourised nicotine products including e-cigarettes with those of tobacco smoke. *Tobacco Control, 27*, 10–17.

Tang MS, Wu X-R, Lee H-W, *et al.* (2019). Electronic-cigarette smoke induces lung adenocarcinoma and bladder urothelial hyperplasia in mice. *Proceedings of the National Academy of Sciences, 116*(43), 21727–21731. doi:10.1073/pnas.1911321116.

Tommasi S, Caliri AW, Caceres A, *et al.* (2019). Deregulation of biologically significant genes and associated molecular pathways in the oral epithelium of electronic cigarette users. *International Journal of Molecular Sciences, 20*, 738.

Chapter 22

Omega-3 Fatty Acids and Cancer Prevention

Omega-3s are predominantly found in fatty fish with fewer amounts in some seeds and nuts (Fig. 1). Most of the studies on Omega-3s have demonstrated protective properties for the heart and brain functions. The animal omega-3 fatty acids include alpha-linolenic acid, eicosapentaenoic acid, and docosahexaenoic acid. These fatty acids also have a very strong anti-inflammatory property and thus provide some health benefits to patients with asthma, cystic fibrosis, colitis, and other chronic diseases. Another interesting property of omega-3 fatty acid is its protection against radiation damages from ultraviolet rays. Although they have been shown to be helpful, higher intake of these fatty acids may result in severe abdominal pains, nausea, cardiac complications as well as diarrhea.

Due to the strong anti-inflammatory properties of omega-3 fatty acids, researchers have suggested they might offer some form of protection against cancer, especially those driven by inflammation such as colorectal, lung, prostate, and liver cancers. Studies have indicated that omega-3 fatty acid decreases tumor-promoting soluble factors such as IL-6 and tumor necrosis factor-alpha without

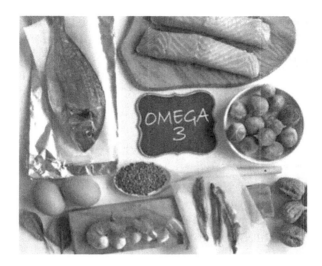

Fig. 1.   Omega-3 fatty acid is derived from meat, seafood, and some vegetables

affecting normal cells, a response that limits the growth of cancer and harnesses the immune system to fight abnormal growth of cells.

In breast cancer studies, omega-3 supplements were associated with the increased expression of tumor suppressors as well as decrease in tumor-supporting signals. Thus, the combinatory effects could limit the growth of breast cancer cells. Although other studies have provided similar findings, more mechanistic studies are needed to reveal the exact mode of action. In prostate cancer cells, omega-3 fatty acids initiated signals that suppress abnormal cell growth and thus provide a novel mechanism for inhibiting cancer cell growth. Other reports have reported that intake of omga-3 fatty acids disrupts the cell membrane of cancer cells, thereby forcing the cells to die. In addition to the individual chemopreventive properties, omega-3 when combined with chemotherapy provide significant improvement in the clinical outcomes of cancer patients.

Using experimental mice, intake of omega-3 resulted in increased expression of tumor-suppressing proteins and decreased expression of tumor-promoting proteins as well as decreased growth and recurrence of colorectal cancer. A much improved outcome was observed when omega-3 was combined with other drugs. A similar mode of action was demonstrated in another independent study where omega-3 but not omega-6 fatty acids were associated with a decrease in the expression of androgen receptor (responsible for the cancer). Understanding the mechanisms of action is key to developing effective dietary therapeutic alternatives for the improvement of patients' survival.

Researchers at the University of Guelph compared the anticancer properties between fish-based and plant-based omega-3 fatty acids on mammary tumors using experimental mice. The type of mammary cancer considered during the experiment was the human epidermal growth factor receptor 2 (HER-2) positive breast cancer that accounts for about 30% of all breast cancers. This type of breast cancer is also considered to be highly aggressive and patients have very poor survival. Upon comparison, the fish-based omega-3 fatty acids showed more potency compared with the plant-based fatty acids. Thus, tumor growth and aggression were reduced in the mice treated with fish-based omega-3 fatty acids by 60–70% compared with those given plant-based omega-3. The rationale behind this study was motivated by the fact that most of the omega-3 fatty acids in the Western countries are derived from plants but not fish. Since this is the first study to demonstrate the difference, more studies are needed to substantiate these findings. However, it will be more beneficial to have moderate proportions of both the plant- and fish-based omega-3 fatty acids.

Regardless, there have been other studies that have either reported weak or no anticancer protection from omega-3 fatty acids. In fact, other reports indicate an association between omega-3 intake and increased risk of prostate cancer. Thus, more studies are still needed to substantiate the cancer preventive properties of omega-3 fatty acids. Although inflammation is central to the development of most cancers, tackling it does not automatically guarantee the absence of cancer. Cancer development goes far beyond inflammation and as such, other factors might contribute to that effect. The addition of moderate amount of omega-3 fatty acids to food might provide some health benefits; however, their anticancer properties might not be guaranteed.

Bibliography

Andreeva VA, Touvier M, Kesse-Guyot E, Julia C, Galan P, Hercberg S. (2012). B Vitamin and/or ω-3 fatty acid supplementation and cancer: Ancillary findings from the supplementation with folate, vitamins b6 and b12, and/or omega-3 fatty acids (SU.FOL.OM3) randomized trial. *Archives of Internal Medicine, 172*(7), 540–547. doi:10.1001/archintern-med.2011.1450.

Berquin IM, Edwards IJ, Chen YQ. (2008). Multi-targeted therapy of cancer by omega-3 fatty acids. *Cancer Letters, 269*(2), 363–377. doi:10.1016/j.canlet.2008.03.044.

Fabian CJ, Kimler BF, Hursting SD. (2015). Omega-3 fatty acids for breast cancer prevention and survivorship. *Breast Cancer Research: BCR, 17*(1), 62. doi:10.1186/s13058-015-0571-6.

Fabian CJ, Kimler BF, Phillips TA, *et al.* (2015). Modulation of breast cancer risk biomarkers by high-dose omega-3 fatty acids: Phase II pilot study in postmenopausal women. *Cancer Prevention Research (Philadelphia, PA.), 8*(10), 922–931. doi:10.1158/1940-6207.CAPR-14-0336.

Freitas R, Campos MM. (2019). Protective effects of omega-3 fatty acids in cancer-related complications. *Nutrients, 11*(5), 945. doi:10.3390/nu11050945.

Friedrichs W, Ruparel SB, Marciniak RA, deGraffenried L. (2011). Omega-3 fatty acid inhibition of prostate cancer progression to hormone independence is associated with suppression of mTOR signaling and androgen receptor expression. *Nutrition and Cancer, 63*(5), 771–777. doi:10.1080/01635581.2011.570892.

Fuentes NR, Kim E, Fan YY, Chapkin RS. (2018). Omega-3 fatty acids, membrane remodeling and cancer prevention. *Molecular Aspects of Medicine, 64*, 79–91. doi:10.1016/j.mam.2018.04.001.

Hawkes JS, Bryan DL, Makrides M, Neumann MA, Gibson RA. (2002). A randomized trial of supplementation with docosahexaenoic acid-rich tuna oil and its effects on the human milk cytokines interleukin 1 beta, interleukin 6, and tumor necrosis factor alpha. *The American Journal of Clinical Nutrition, 75*, 754–760.

Holm T, Berge RK, Andreassen AK, *et al.* (2001). Omega-3 fatty acids enhance tumor necrosis factor-alpha levels in heart transplant recipients. *Transplantation, 72*, 706–711.

Laviano A, Rianda S, Molfino A, Rossi F. (2013). Omega-3 fatty acids in cancer. *Current Opinion in Clinical Nutrition and Metabolic Care, 16*(2), 156–161. doi:10.1097/MCO.0b013e32835d2d99.

Liu J, Abdelmagid SA, Pinelli CJ, *et al.* (2017). Marine fish oil is more potent than plant-based n-3 polyunsaturated fatty acids in the prevention of mammary tumors. *The Journal of Nutritional Biochemistry, 55,* 41–52. doi:10.1016/j.jnutbio.2017.12.011.

Liu Z, Hopkins MM, Zhang Z, *et al.* (2015). Omega-3 fatty acids and other FFA4 agonists inhibit growth factor signaling in human prostate cancer cells. *The Journal of Pharmacology and Experimental Therapeutics, 352*(2), 380–394. doi:10.1124/jpet.114.218974.

Murphy RA, Mourtzakis M, Chu QS, Baracos VE, Reiman T, Mazurak VC. (2011). Nutritional intervention with fish oil provides a benefit over standard of care for weight and skeletal muscle mass in patients with non-small cell lung cancer receiving chemotherapy. *Cancer, 117*(8), 1775–1782.

Vasudevan A, Yu Y, Banerjee S, *et al.* (2014). Omega-3 fatty acid is a potential preventive agent for recurrent colon cancer. *Cancer Prevention Research (Philadelphia, PA.), 7*(11), 1138–1148. doi:10.1158/1940-6207. CAPR-14-0177.

Weiss G, Meyer F, Matthies B, Pross M, Koenig W, Lippert H. (2002). Immunomodulation by perioperative administration of n-3 fatty acids. *The British Journal of Nutrition, 87*(Suppl. 1), S89–S94.

Chapter 23

Birth Control and Cancer Risk

Oral contraceptives, also known as birth control pills, contain synthetic forms of natural female hormones — estrogen and progesterone (Fig. 1). They are used mainly to prevent conception or pregnancy and usually administered orally. Birth control basically works by preventing the sperms from entering the womb as well as suppressing ovulation. Beside the oral administering of contraceptives, there are other methods such as skin implant, injection, patch, and vaginal ring insertion. Although the method of delivery might differ, their mode of action is mostly the same. There are other benefits of birth controls other than preventing unplanned pregnancies. They help suppress or reduce menstrual cramps and bleeding during menstruation and ovulation. They also help in the management of side effects of excessive male hormone production as well as reducing the risks of developing uterine and ovarian cancers.

Studies on the link between birth control and cancer have mostly been conducted on orally administered pills. Most of these studies are largely observational studies that cannot provide causality or establish a mechanistic link between pills and cancer development or risk. Notwithstanding, consistent evidence has shown that women who mostly use oral pills are at a higher risk of

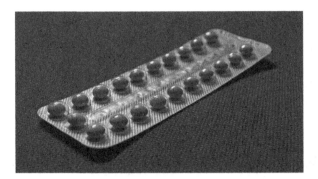

Fig. 1.   Birth control pills

developing breast and cervical cancers. However, in this same cohort of women, the risk for developing ovarian, endometrial, and colorectal cancers is reduced.

The protection against ovarian and endometrial cancers is a result of reduced ovulation, which also minimizes the exposure of the body to hormonal secretions. This could offer up to 25 years of protection after taking the pills for five years and also reduce ovarian cancer risk by half, whereas the risk of endometrial cancers could persist for almost 10 years. The protection is effective such that even women with BRCA genetic mutations could benefit from it. Increasing evidence has shown that women using orally administered pills stand to benefit from protection against ovarian and endometrial cancers; however, the exact mechanism is yet to be unveiled. Understanding the mechanism could hold the key to developing novel therapeutic approaches to fighting cancer.

Nonetheless, there have been studies that have shown a consistent link between other types of cancers and oral pills. In large epidemiological studies, researchers demonstrated that women who use oral pills have 7% increased risk of developing breast cancer compared with nonusers. This risk was, however, reduced when these women stopped using the pills. In a study involving about 116,000 nurses, breast cancer risk was seen to be higher in those who used a particular pill called triphasic. This increase in breast cancer risk was also reported in another study where the women used the triphasic pill formulations. In a Danish study, women who used oral pills had 20% increase in breast cancer risk compared with those who did not use them. Researchers detected that the risk is dependent on the type of pill formulations taken by the women.

The number of years a woman uses oral pills will determine her risk of developing cervical cancer. Using oral pills for less than five years has a modest increase in cervical cancer risk. However, more than five years of usage could increase a woman's risk to about 80%. Although this sounds alarming, the risk decreases after women halt the usage. In most cases, cervical cancers are caused by human papillomavirus (HPV) infection that is transmitted sexually. Thus, HPV negative women are unlikely to develop cervical cancer regardless of her using oral pills. More studies are, however, needed to further strengthen the link between cervical cancer development and orally administered pills.

Unlike oral pills, there are very few studies on other contraceptives such as IUD and cancer association. Researchers should invest more time into investigating other methods of contraception. The association of cancer and contraceptives is still not clear since most of the studies are either for or against the link. This should not scare women who have no option but to use oral contraceptives. The best way out is to have a candid discussion with your health practitioner about the best contraceptive with minimal risks.

Bibliography

Bassuk SS, Manson JE. (2015). Oral contraceptives and menopausal hormone therapy: Relative and attributable risks of cardiovascular disease, cancer, and other health outcomes. *Annals of Epidemiology, 25*(3), 193–200.

Beaber EF, Buist DS, Barlow WE, Malone KE, Reed SD, Li CI. (2014). Recent oral contraceptive use by formulation and breast cancer risk among women 20 to 49 years of age. *Cancer Research, 74*(15), 4078–4089.

Bhupathiraju SN, Grodstein F, Stampfer MJ, Willett WC, Hu FB, Manson JE. (2016). Exogenous hormone use: Oral contraceptives, postmenopausal hormone therapy, and health outcomes in the Nurses' Health Study. *American Journal of Public Health, 106*(9), 1631–1637.

Burkman R, Schlesselman JJ, Zieman M. (2004). Safety concerns and health benefits associated with oral contraception. *American Journal of Obstetrics and Gynecology, 190*(Suppl. 4), S5–22.

Collaborative Group on Epidemiological Studies on Endometrial Cancer. (2015). Endometrial cancer and oral contraceptives: An individual participant meta-analysis of 27 276 women with endometrial cancer from 36 epidemiological studies. *Lancet Oncology, 16*(9), 1061–1070.

Collaborative Group on Hormonal Factors in Breast Cancer. (1996). Breast cancer and hormonal contraceptives: Collaborative reanalysis of individual data on 53,297 women with breast cancer and 100,239 women without breast cancer from 54 epidemiological studies. *Lancet, 347*(9017), 1713–1727.

Friebel TM, Domchek SM, Rebbeck TR. (2014). Modifiers of cancer risk in BRCA1 and BRCA2 mutation carriers: Systematic review and meta-analysis. *Journal of the National Cancer Institute, 106*(6), dju091.

Gierisch JM, Coeytaux RR, Urrutia RP, *et al.* (2013). Oral contraceptive use and risk of breast, cervical, colorectal, and endometrial cancers: A systematic review. *Cancer Epidemiology, Biomarkers & Prevention, 22*(11), 1931–1943.

Havrilesky LJ, Moorman PG, Lowery WJ, *et al.* (2013). Oral contraceptive pills as primary prevention for ovarian cancer: A systematic review and meta-analysis. *Obstetrics and Gynecology, 122*(1), 139–147.

Hunter DJ, Colditz GA, Hankinson SE, *et al.* (2010). Oral contraceptive use and breast cancer: A prospective study of young women. *Cancer Epidemiology Biomarkers and Prevention, 19*(10), 2496–2502.

IARC Working Group on the Evaluation of Carcinogenic Risks to Humans. (2012). Pharmaceuticals. Combined estrogen-progestogen contraceptivesExit disclaimer. *IARC Monographs on the Evaluation of Carcinogenic Risks to Humans, 100A*, 283–311.

International Collaboration of Epidemiological Studies of Cervical Cancer, Appleby P, Beral V, *et al.* (2007). Cervical cancer and hormonal contraceptives: Collaborative reanalysis of individual data for 16,573 women with cervical cancer and 35,509 women without cervical cancer from 24 epidemiological studies. *Lancet, 370*(9599), 1609–1621.

Iodice S, Barile M, Rotmensz N, *et al.* (2010). Oral contraceptive use and breast or ovarian cancer risk in BRCA1/2 carriers: A meta-analysis. *European Journal of Cancer, 46*(12), 2275–2284.

Iversen L, Sivasubramaniam S, Lee AJ, Fielding S, Hannaford PC. (2017). Lifetime cancer risk and combined oral contraceptives: The royal college of general practitioners' oral contraception study. *American Journal of Obstetrics and Gynecology, 216*(6), 580.e1–580.e9.

Luan NN, Wu L, Gong TT, Wang YL, Lin B, Wu QJ. (2015). Nonlinear reduction in risk for colorectal cancer by oral contraceptive use: A meta-analysis of epidemiological studies. *Cancer Causes & Control, 26*(1), 65–78.

Michels KA, Pfeiffer RM, Brinton LA, Trabert B. (2018). Modification of the associations between duration of oral contraceptive use and ovarian, endometrial, breast, and colorectal cancers. *JAMA Oncology, 4*, 516–521. doi:10.1001/jamaoncol.2017.4942.

Moorman PG, Havrilesky LJ, Gierisch JM, *et al.* (2013). Oral contraceptives and risk of ovarian cancer and breast cancer among high-risk women: A systematic review and meta-analysis. *Journal of Clinical Oncology, 31*(33), 4188–4198.

Mørch LS, Skovlund CW, Hannaford PC, Iversen L, Fielding S, Lidegaard Ø. (2017). Contemporary hormonal contraception and the risk of breast cancer. *New England Journal of Medicine, 377*(23), 2228–2239.

Murphy N, Xu L, Zervoudakis A, *et al.* (2017). Reproductive and menstrual factors and colorectal cancer incidence in the Women's Health Initiative Observational Study. *British Journal of Cancer, 116*(1), 117–125.

Roura E, Travier N, Waterboer T, *et al.* (2016). The influence of hormonal factors on the risk of developing cervical cancer and pre-cancer: Results from the EPIC Cohort. *PLoS One, 11*(1), e0147029.

Smith JS, Green J, Berrington de Gonzalez A, *et al.* (2003). Cervical cancer and use of hormonal contraceptives: A systematic review. *Lancet, 361*(9364), 1159–1167.

Wentzensen N, Berrington de Gonzalez A. (2015). The Pill's gestation: From birth control to cancer prevention. *Lancet Oncology, 16*(9), 1004–1006. doi:10.1016/S1470-2045(15)00211-9.

Wentzensen N, Poole EM, Trabert B, *et al.* (2016). Ovarian cancer risk factors by histologic subtype: An analysis from the Ovarian Cancer Cohort Consortium. *Journal of Clinical Oncology, 34*(24), 2888–2898.

Chapter 24

Do Viruses, Parasites, and Bacteria Cause Cancer?

Cancer is said to be the manifestation of several disorders happening at the same time in the body. There are several risk factors that predispose a person to cancer: activation of tumor-promoting genes, inhibition of tumor-suppressing genes, weak immune system, family history, and many more. Rarely will you hear about the possibilities that viral, bacterial, and parasitic infections cause cancer. The answer is YES, there are some infections that can create a suitable environment for the development of cancer. There are viruses and bacteria that interfere with the signals that keep cell growth under check (Fig. 1). Also, they have the ability to suppress the immune system as well as cause chronic inflammation, responses that are favorable for the development of colitis-associated cancers. When the immune system is suppressed or shut down, cells grow uncontrollably without any check. Thus, cancer cells have the upper hand to spread to other parts of the body and cause more harm. At this stage, treatment becomes difficult and patients have poor prognosis. Most of these infections are transmitted from person to person via blood, body fluids, sharing of needle, and having unprotected sex.

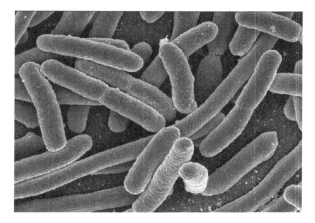

Fig. 1. Highly magnified bacteria by a powerful microscope

Liver cancer, for instance, could be caused by chronic infections with hepatitis B and C viruses. These viruses could be transferred from mother to child during delivery and that automatically puts the baby at risk of developing liver cancer. Vaccination against this infection is a sure way of escaping liver cancers mediated by hepatitis B and C viruses. In a study conducted with participants from different ethnic backgrounds, it was observed that hepatitis B-mediated liver cancer was mostly seen among patients from African and Asian backgrounds. These patients were older than 40 years and had at least a family member suffering from liver cancer. This was independent of whether the patients had cirrhosis or not. It is therefore recommended that most liver cancer patients are screened for hepatic viral infections. In a Danish nationwide study, it was observed that the hepatitis B patients were 17-fold higher at risk of developing liver cancer compared with those without the viral infection.

Cervical cancer is mainly caused by the infection of human papillomavirus (HPV). Other studies have shown that aside from cervical cancer, HPV also causes vaginal, penile, anal, and vulvar cancers which are, however, less commonly diagnosed. HPV vaccine is one of the most successful stories ever in the history of medicine and has provided lots of benefits to most people especially females.

In many countries, ladies at very young ages are vaccinated and this has contributed to the success story. Aside from genital-related cancers, HPV type 16 is also detected in most patients with cancers of the oropharynx and oral cavity. The transfer of the virus from the genital area to the mouth could possibly be due to oral sex and other sexual engagements.

Gastric cancer is another type of cancer that could be caused by bacteria known as *Helicobacter pylori* (*H. pylori*). One is usually infected upon consuming contaminated food or water. It is interesting to note that about two-thirds of the world's population carries *H. pylori*. The infection rate is, however, higher in the developing nations compared with the developed countries. The bacteria are able to activate tumor-promoting pathways in epithelial cells and enable the cells to divide uncontrollably. Chronic inflammation due to infection results in the production of soluble chemicals that maintain the bacterial composition and numbers in the gut. The *H. pylori* take advantage of this system to thrive and elicit more damage to neighboring cells. *H. pylori* also have the ability to silence tumor-suppressing genes by a unique mechanism called hypermethylation, an effect that suppresses the functions of genes responsible for fighting cancer development.

In Africa and other developing countries, most bladder cancer patients are infested with parasitic worms. These worms enter via the skin and then the bladder. People living with HIV are also at high risk for some types of cancers such as lymphomas, Hodgkin and non-Hodgkin lymphomas, Kaposi sarcoma, and others. The HIV suppresses the immune system and thus contributes to the aggressiveness of cancer. Additionally, Epstein–Barr virus (EBV), human T-cell leukemia/lymphoma virus type 1 (HTLV-1), and Merkel cell polyomavirus (MCPyV) infections are highly associated with lymphomas, adult T-cell leukemia/lymphoma, and Merkel cell carcinoma (a rare form of skin cancer), respectively.

Regular screening for viral infections could eliminate some of these cancers as well as protect partners or close relatives since most of these are contagious. Most often, there are effective medications for the treatment of these infections. Discussing with your healthcare practitioner will be of great benefit since they are well trained to recommend the best diagnostic or therapeutic options for your wellness.

Bibliography

Andersen ES, Omland LH, Jepsen P, *et al.* (2015). Risk of all-type cancer, hepatocellular carcinoma, non-Hodgkin lymphoma and pancreatic cancer in patients infected with hepatitis B virus. *Journal of Viral Hepatitis, 22*(10), 828–834. doi:10.1111/jvh.12391.

Anttila T, Saikku P, Koskela P, *et al.* (2001). Serotypes of Chlamydia trachomatis and risk for development of cervical squamous cell carcinoma. *JAMA, 285,* 47–51.

Armstrong GL, Wasley A, Simard EP, *et al.* (2006). The prevalence of Hepatitis C Virus infection in the United States, 1999 through 2002. *Annals of Internal Medicine, 144,* 705–714.

Ault KA. (2006). Epidemiology and natural history of human papillomavirus infections in the female genital tract. *Infectious Diseases in Obstetrics and Gynecology, 2006*(Suppl), 40470.

Bhatia A, Burtness B. (2015). Human papillomavirus-associated oropharyngeal cancer: Defining risk groups and clinical trials. *Journal of Clinical Oncology: Official Journal of the American Society of Clinical Oncology, 33*(29), 3243–3250. doi:10.1200/JCO.2015.61.2358.

Bialasiewicz S, Lambert SB, Whiley DM, Nissen MD, Sloots TP. (2009). Merkel cell polyomavirus DNA in respiratory specimens from children and adults. *Emerging Infectious Diseases, 15*(3), 492–494.

Bonnet F, Lewden C, May T, *et al.* (2004). Malignancy-related causes of death in human immunodeficiency virus-infected patients in the era of highly active antiretroviral therapy. *Cancer, 101,* 317–324.

Borges JD, Souza VA, Giambartolomei C, *et al.* (2012). Transmission of human herpesvirus type 8 infection within families in American indigenous populations from the Brazilian Amazon. *The Journal of Infectious Disease, 205,* 1869–1876.

Brown LM. (2000). *Helicobacter pylori*: Epidemiology and routes of transmission. *Epidemiologic Reviews, 22,* 283–297.

Buchschacher GL Jr, Wong-Staal F. (2011). RNA viruses. In DeVita VT, Lawrence TS, Rosenberg SA (Eds.), *Cancer: Principles & practice of oncology* (9th ed., pp. 186–192). Philadelphia, PA: Lippincott Williams & Wilkins.

Caskey MF, Morgan DJ, Porto AF, *et al.* (2007). Clinical manifestations associated with HTLV type I infection: A cross-sectional study. *AIDS Research and Human Retroviruses, 23,* 365–371.

Centers for Disease Control and Prevention. (2010). HIV transmission through transfusion — Missouri and Colorado, 2008. *MMWR. Morbidity and Mortality Weekly Report, 59*(41), 1335–1339.

Centers for Disease Control and Prevention. (2014a). Hepatitis B information for health professionals. Retrieved on December 11, 2019.

Centers for Disease Control and Prevention. (2014b). Hepatitis C information for health professionals. Retrieved on December 11, 2019.

Chayanupatkul M, Omino R, Mittal S, *et al.* (2017). Hepatocellular carcinoma in the absence of cirrhosis in patients with chronic hepatitis B virus infection. *Journal of Hepatology, 66*(2), 355–362. doi:10.1016/j.jhep.2016.09.013.

Chen AA, Gheit T, Franceschi S, Tommasino M, Clifford GM, IARC HPV Variant Study Group. (2015). Human papillomavirus 18 genetic variation and cervical cancer risk worldwide. *Journal of Virology, 89*(20), 10680–10687. doi:10.1128/JVI.01747-15.

Chen T, Hedman L, Mattila PS. (2011). Serological evidence of Merkel cell polyomavirus primary infections in childhood. *Journal of Clinical Virology: The Official Publication of the Pan American Society for Clinical Virology, 50,* 125–129.

Chen T, Hudnall SD. (2006). Anatomical mapping of human herpesvirus reservoirs of infection. *Modern Pathology, 19,* 726–737.

Cheng AS, Li MS, Kang W, *et al.* (2013). *Helicobacter pylori* causes epigenetic dysregulation of FOXD3 to promote gastric carcinogenesis. *Gastroenterology, 144*(1), 122–133.e9. doi:10.1053/j.gastro.2012.10.002.

Cote TR, Biggar RJ, Rosenberg PS, *et al.* (1997). Non-Hodgkin's lymphoma among people with AIDS: Incidence, presentation and public health burden. *International Journal of Cancer, 73,* 645–650.

Engels EA, Atkinson JO, Graubard BI, *et al.* (2007). Risk factors for human herpesvirus 8 infection among adults in the United States and evidence for sexual transmission. *The Journal of Infectious Diseases, 196,* 199–207.

Feng H, Shuda M, Chang Y, Moore PS. (2008). Clonal integration of a polyomavirus in human Merkel cell carcinoma. *Science, 319,* 1096–1100.

Herrero R, Castellsagué X, Pawlita M, *et al.* (2003). For the IARC multicenter oral cancer study group, human papillomavirus and oral cancer: The international agency for research on cancer multicenter study. *JNCI: Journal of the National Cancer Institute, 95*(23), 1772–1783. doi:10.1093/jnci/djg107

Heymann DL. (Ed.). (2008). *Control of communicable diseases manual* (19th ed., pp. 393–402). Washington, DC: American Public Health Association.

Holzinger F, Z'graggen K, Buchler MW. (1999). Mechanisms of biliary carcinogenesis: A pathogenetic multi-stage cascade towards cholangiocarcinoma. *Annals of Oncology: Official Journal of the European Society for Medical Oncology/ESMO, 10*, 122–126.

Howley PM, Ganem D, Kieff E. (2011). DNA Viruses. In DeVita VT, Lawrence TS, Rosenberg SA (Eds.), *Cancer: Principles & practice of oncology* (9th ed., pp. 173–185). Philadelphia: Lippincott Williams & Wilkins.

IARC Monographs on the Evaluation of Carcinogenic Risks to Humans. (2012). Volume 100B: A Review of human carcinogens: Biological agents. *International Agency for Research on Cancer.* Retrieved on December 11, 2019.

Johnson KS, Ottemann KM. (2018). Colonization, localization, and inflammation: The roles of *H. pylori* chemotaxis in vivo. *Current Opinion in Microbiology, 41*, 51–57. doi:10.1016/j.mib.2017.11.019.

Lambert PF, Sugden B. (2014). Chapter 11: Viruses and human cancer. In Niederhuber JE, Armitage JO, Dorshow JH, Kastan MB, Tepper JE (Eds.), *Abeloff's Clinical Oncology* (5th ed.). Philadelphia, PA: Elsevier.

Lanoy E, Dores GM, Madeleine MM, Toro JR, Fraumeni JF, Engels EA. (2009). Epidemiology of nonkeratinocytic skin cancers among persons with AIDS in the United States. *AIDS, 23*, 385–393.

Li WQ, Ma JL, Zhang L, *et al.* (2014). Effects of *Helicobacter pylori* treatment on gastric cancer incidence and mortality in subgroups. *Journal of the National Cancer Institute, 106*(7), dju116. doi:10.1093/jnci/dju116.

Manfredi JJ, Dong J, Liu WJ, *et al.* (2005). Evidence against a role for SV40 in human mesothelioma. *Cancer Research, 65*, 2602–2609.

Mork J, Lie AK, Glattre E, *et al.* (2001). Human papillomavirus infection as a risk factor for squamous-cell carcinoma of the head and neck. *The New England Journal of Medicine, 344*, 1125–1131.

Nagachinta T, Duerr A, Suriyanon V, *et al.* (1997). Risk factors for HIV-1 transmission from HIV-seropositive male blood donors to their regular female partners in northern Thailand. *AIDS, 11*, 1765–1772.

National Cancer Institute. (2011). HIV infection and cancer risk. Retrieved on 2019, December 11.

National Cancer Institute. (2012). HPV and cancer. Retrieved on 2019, December 11.

National Cancer Institute. (2013). *Helicobacter pylori* and cancer. Retrieved on December 11, 2019.

National Cancer Institute. Simian virus 40 and human cancer: Fact sheet. Retrieved on December 11, 2019.

National Cancer Institute. Studies find no evidence that SV40 is related to human cancer. Retrieved on December 11, 2019.

Poiesz BJ, Papsidero LD, Ehrlich G, *et al.* (2001). Prevalence of HTLV-I-associated T-cell lymphoma. *American Journal of Hematology, 66*, 32–38.

Qu L, Jenkins F, Triulzi DJ. (2010). Human herpesvirus 8 genomes and seroprevalence in United States blood donors. *Transfusion, 50*, 1050–1056.

Rodig SJ, Cheng J, Wardzala J, *et al.* (2012). Improved detection suggests all Merkel cell carcinomas harbor Merkel polyomavirus. *The Journal of Clinical Investigation, 122*, 4645–4653.

Sahasrabuddhe VV, Shiels MS, McGlynn KA, Engels EA. (2012). The risk of hepatocellular carcinoma among individuals with acquired immuno-deficiency syndrome in the United States. *Cancer, 118*, 6226–6233.

Wroblewski LE, Piazuelo MB, Chaturvedi R, *et al.* (2015). *Helicobacter pylori* targets cancer-associated apical-junctional constituents in gastroids and gastric epithelial cells. *Gut, 64*(5), 720–730. doi:10.1136/gutjnl-2014-307650.

Chapter 25

Tobacco Smoking Increases Your Risk of Cancer

Smoking of tobacco is a serious health concern (Fig. 1). Regardless of the health warnings, people still indulge in tobacco smoking. Tobacco contains a plethora of very harmful chemicals. The smoke generated by smoking is known to contain over 7,000 chemicals with at least 250 known to be harmful to the health of the smokers and nonsmokers (passive smokers). About 70 out of 250 of these known harmful substances are classified as cancer-causing agents. Examples of these cancer-causing chemicals are arsenic, benzene, cumene, ethylene oxide, formaldehyde, acetaldehyde, nickel, vinyl chloride, polycyclic aromatic hydrocarbons (PAHs), polonium-210, and beryllium.

One would think that smoking only affects the smoker and his/ her lungs. However, there is more to that. The chemicals from tobacco are able to move via your blood and affect the entire body and cause other types of cancers. Standing close to a smoker can also predispose you to cancer-causing chemicals once inhaled. Such people are called passive smokers. Stopping smoking is key to avoiding health disasters associated with tobacco. Continual smoking creates damages beyond the body's repairing capacity, thus, serving as a fertile ground for the development of cancer.

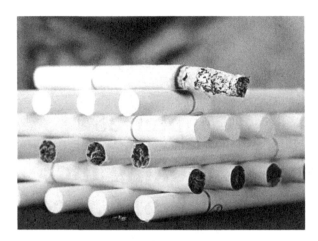

Fig. 1. Cigarettes (tobacco) on display

Unlike other risk factors, the link between smoking and cancer is well proven and established beyond doubt. Reports indicate that smoking is the cause of 15 types of cancers including lung cancers. Seven out of ten lung cancer cases are attributed to excessive smoking and smoking is the most common cause of cancer death worldwide. Smoking-related cancers include liver, bladder, bowel, kidney, mouth, upper throat, lung, nose, esophagus, cervical, and stomach cancers. Leukemia and other heart complications are also well documented. The more cigarettes one smokes, the higher the risk of developing cancer. Smoking 15 cigarettes have the ability to cause DNA damage that results in the cell becoming cancerous. Thus, reducing the frequency and the number of cigarettes has the potential to reduce cancer risk.

Aside from the cancer-causing properties of tobacco, combining smoking with alcohol is a next-level deadly combination whose detrimental effects are more than either of them. Mouth and upper throat cancers are predominant in people who combine both tobacco smoking and alcohol drinking. Alcohol has the ability to increase the rate at which tobacco chemicals are assimilated into the blood. The fact is there is no tobacco product that is safe regardless of the medium of usage. Pipes, cigars, bidis, kreteks, and water pipes are all forms of tobacco products that have very strong association with cancer risk. Cigars contain more harmful chemicals than cigarette smoke and can cause lung, larynx, mouth, and esophageal cancers. Bidis is mainly popular in India, which is a flavored cigarette rolled in a dried leaf. Bidis is associated with cancers of the mouth, lung, throat, and esophagus. There have also been reports of heart complications in users. Pipe, another tobacco product that is mostly used in the Asian and African regions, increases cancer risk and is also associated with cancers of the mouth and gut. All these findings point to the fact that there is no safety when it comes to tobacco usage regardless of how it is used.

Apart from cigarette, there are other forms of tobacco that are smokeless but also very harmful. Examples are spit tobacco, chewing tobacco, oral tobacco, dissolvable tobacco, and snuff. These forms of tobacco products are significantly associated with cancers of the mouth, esophagus, and pancreas. In situations where a person is diagnosed with tobacco-smoking cancer, quitting smoking could help improve the prognosis of the patient as well as reduce the risk of dying by 40%. Quitting smoking also reduces the chances of having other cancer-related complications and helps improve the efficacy of treatments. Tobacco addiction is very difficult to deal with; hence addicts should get support from counselors or experienced healthcare professionals who could take them through medically recommended guidelines to help them deal with their addictions.

Bibliography

Austoni E, Mirone V, Parazzini F, *et al.* (2005). Smoking as a risk factor for erectile dysfunction: Data from the Andrology Prevention Weeks 2001–2002. A study of the Italian Society of Andrology (S.I.A.). *European Urology, 48*(5), 810–818.

Brown KF, Rumgay H, Dunlop C, *et al.* (2018). The fraction of cancer attributable to modifiable risk factors in England, Wales, Scotland, Northern Ireland, and the United Kingdom in 2015. *British Journal of Cancer, 118*, 1130–1141.

Cancer Research UK. Lung cancer statistics. Retrieved on December 12, 2019 from Cruk.org/health-professional/cancer-statistics/statistics-by-cancer-type/lung-cancer.

Cobb C, Ward KD, Maziak W, Shihadeh AL, Eissenberg T. (2010). Waterpipe tobacco smoking: An emerging health crisis in the United States. *American Journal of Health Behavior, 34*(3), 275–285.

Corey CG, Ambrose BK, Apelberg BJ, King, BA. (2015). Flavored tobacco product use among middle and high school students — United States, 2014. *Morbidity and Mortality Weekly Report, 64*(38), 1066–1070.

Flanders WD, Lally CA, Zhu BP, Henley SJ, Thun MJ. (2003). Lung cancer mortality in relation to age, duration of smoking, and daily cigarette consumption: Results from cancer prevention study II. *Cancer Research, 63*, 6556–6562.

Gandini S, Botteri E, Iodice S, *et al.* (2008). Tobacco smoking and cancer: A meta-analysis. *International Journal of Cancer, 1*, 155–164.

Hatsukami DK, Stead LF, Gupta PC. (2008). Tobacco addiction. *Lancet, 371*(9629), 2027–2038.

Hecht SS. (2003). Tobacco carcinogens, their biomarkers and tobacco-induced cancer. *Nature Reviews, 3*(10), 733–744.

Henley SJ, Thun MJ, Chao A, Calle EE. (2004). Association between exclusive pipe smoking and mortality from cancer and other diseases. *Journal of the National Cancer Institute, 96*(11), 853–861.

Inoue-Choi M, Hartge P, Liao LM, Caporaso N, Freedman ND. (2018). Association between long-term low-intensity cigarette smoking and incidence of smoking-related cancer in the National Institutes of Health-AARP cohort. *International Journal of Cancer, 142*(2), 271–280.

Inoue-Choi M, Liao LM, Reyes-Guzman C, Hartge P, Caporaso N, Freedman ND. (2017). Association of long-term, low-intensity smoking with all-cause and cause-specific mortality in the National Institutes of Health-AARP diet and health study. *JAMA Internal Medicine, 177*(1), 87–95.

International Agency for Research on Cancer. (2004). Tobacco smoke and involuntary smoking. *IARC Monographs on the Evaluation of Carcinogenic Risks to Humans, 83*, 1–1413.

International Agency for Research on Cancer. (2007). *Smokeless Tobacco and Some Tobacco-Specific N-Nitrosamines*, Vol. 89.

Jha P, Ramasundarahettige C, Landsman V, *et al.* (2013). 21st-century hazards of smoking and benefits of cessation in the United States. *New England Journal of Medicine, 368*(4), 341–350.

Knishkowy B, Amitai Y. (2005). Water-pipe (narghile) smoking: An emerging health risk behavior. *Pediatrics, 116*(1), e113–119.

McBride CM, Ostroff JS. (2003). Teachable moments for promoting smoking cessation: The context of cancer care and survivorship. *Cancer Control, 10*(4), 325–333.

Nash SH, Liao LM, Harris TB, Freedman ND. (2017). Cigarette smoking and mortality in adults aged 70 years and older: Results from the NIH-AARP cohort. *American Journal of Preventive Medicine, 52*(3), 276–283.

National Cancer Institute. (2017, January). *Cancer trends progress report: Second-hand smoke exposure.* Bethesda, MD: National Institutes of Health, U.S. Department of Health and Human Services.

National Toxicology Program. (2016). Tobacco-related exposures. In Report on Carcinogens. Fourteenth Edition. U.S. Department of Health and Human Services, Public Health Service, National Toxicology Program.

Parsons A, Daley A, Begh R, Aveyard P. (2010). Influence of smoking cessation after diagnosis of early stage lung cancer on prognosis: Systematic review of observational studies with meta-analysis. *British Medical Journal, 340*, b5569.

Peto R, Darby S, Deo H, Silcocks P, Whitley E, Doll R. (2000). Smoking, smoking cessation, and lung cancer in the U.K. since 1950: Combination of national statistics with two case-control studies. *British Medical Journal, 321*(7257), 323–329.

Piano MR, Benowitz NL, Fitzgerald GA, *et al.* (2010). Impact of smokeless tobacco products on cardiovascular disease: Implications for policy, prevention, and treatment: A policy statement from the American Heart Association. *Circulation, 122*(15), 1520–1544. doi:10.1161/CIR.0b013e3181f432c3.

Prignot JJ, Sasco AJ, Poulet E, Gupta PC, Aditama TY. (2008). Alternative forms of tobacco use. *International Journal of Tuberculosis and Lung Disease, 12*(7), 718–727.

Smith-Simone S, Maziak W, Ward KD, Eissenberg T. (2008). Waterpipe tobacco smoking: Knowledge, attitudes, beliefs, and behavior in two U.S. samples. *Nicotine Tobacco Research, 10*(2), 393–398.

Travis LB, Rabkin CS, Brown LM, *et al.* (2006). Cancer survivorship-genetic susceptibility and second primary cancers: Research strategies and recommendations. *Journal of the National Cancer Institute, 98*(1), 15–25.

U.S. Department of Health and Human Services. (1990). *The health benefits of smoking cessation: A report of the surgeon general.* Rockville, MD: U.S. Department of Health and Human Services, Public Health Service,

Centers for Disease Control, Center for Chronic Disease Prevention and Health Promotion, Office on Smoking and Health.

U.S. Environmental Protection Agency. (1992). *Respiratory health effects of passive smoking: Lung cancer and other disorders.* Washington, DC: U.S. Environmental Protection Agency, Office of Health and Environmental Assessment, Office of Research and Development.

Villanti AC, Richardson A, Vallone DM, Rath JM. (2013). Flavored tobacco product use among U.S. young adults. *American Journal of Preventive Medicine, 44*(4), 388–391.

Walter V, Jansen L, Hoffmeister M, Brenner H. (2014). Smoking and survival of colorectal cancer patients: Systematic review and meta-analysis. *Annals of Oncology, 25*(8), 1517–1525.

Warren GW, Kasza KA, Reid ME, Cummings KM, Marshall JR. (2013). Smoking at diagnosis and survival in cancer patients. *International Journal of Cancer, 132*(2), 401–410.

Wyss A, Hashibe M, Chuang SC, *et al.* (2013). Cigarette, cigar, and pipe smoking and the risk of head and neck cancers: Pooled analysis in the international head and neck cancer epidemiology consortium. *American Journal of Epidemiology, 178*(5), 679–690.

Chapter 26

Do Food Supplements Treat Cancer?

Food supplements contain one or more dietary ingredients that are usually taken orally to achieve high levels of micronutrients compared with that gotten from diet alone. There are lots of food supplements currently available in the market and these could be purchased without any prescription. Most of these supplements contain minerals, herbs, amino acids, enzymes, vitamins, and botanicals that could be packaged as powder, liquid, pills, tablets, and capsules. Although food supplements are meant to meet the daily requirements of nutrients needed by the body, some people use them for various reasons including body building, relaxation, sexual pleasure, and overall health (Fig. 1).

For a while now, most of the manufacturers of these supplements make wild claims about the anticancer properties of their products, although they provide limited evidence to that effect. With the exception of the role of calcium in fighting colon cancer, there is no approved food supplement meant to be used for the treatment of cancer. Most of these supplements are unregulated and the claims they put out there are deceptive. Although most of these vitamins and minerals could have a positive impact in the overall

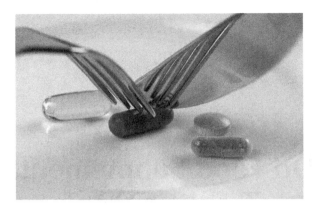

Fig. 1.   Dietary supplements

health status of a person, their anticancer properties have not yet been proven. Nonetheless, these manufacturers make advertisements suggestive of the fact that their products could be used to treat or cure cancer. These statements are false until proven with scientific evidence as well as approved by the FDA. Until then, food supplements are generally not anticancer products but could offer general health benefits.

It is important to note that most of the advertisements of these supplements are based on personal experiences also known as anecdotal evidence. Thus, such evidence lacks objectivity and mechanistic research findings. The food supplement industry is gradually becoming a moneymaking venture where wild claims are mostly made without any scientific evidence to win the trust of customers. There are businessmen who purposely go into such businesses for the financial gain but not the health benefits they bring. One of the reasons why these products are all over the place is that food supplements do not necessarily require approval from the FDA for them to be marketed. Also, no clinical trials are needed before the products are marketed. However, the FDA makes sure any product that comes to the market is safe and does not cause any harmful effect to the users. As to whether these supplements work or not is not the responsibility of the FDA. Apart from making sure these products are safe, the FDA also insists the right claims are made about food supplements and correct labels are provided by the manufacturers. One difficulty is that the FDA is limited and cannot review all food supplements being channeled out into the market and thus, most of these industries take advantage of it to make false claims. There have been instances where the FDA has halted the sales of some products due to false claims, safety reasons, or wrong labeling of products.

It is important to note that some supplements such as folic acid can help reduce the risk of certain diseases but they are in no way intended to cure, treat, diagnose, or relieve the effects of diseases. The moment an industry claims a food supplement can do what prescribed medicines can do, there is a cause for alarm right there. It is either the supplement contains an unapproved chemical or the claims are false. The false advertisements by some of these supplement makers have ended the lives of people. There are instances where people fell for these advertisements and stopped taking their prescribed medications.

Depending on a patient's condition, taking food supplements should be done in consultation with his or her doctor. Most of these dietary supplements might interfere with chemotherapy and other cancer drugs and make the situation of the patient even worse. In no way should cancer patients replace their prescribed medicines with food supplements. Also, patients should be candid with their doctors on the type of supplements they are taking so as to help in their treatment management. In some cases, doctors may recommend the use of specific food supplements alongside the main treatments to help with loss of appetite, injuries from radiation, and mouth sores.

The US FDA reports that 1,009 cases of adverse effects were documented in 2010. The number keeps increasing as the cases reported in 2011 and 2012 were 2,047 and 2,844, respectively. It is estimated that this number could reach 10,000 by the year 2020 if care is not taken to curb the situation. It is not illegal to purchase food supplements; however, care should be taken when buying them. Open discussions with your healthcare provider will go a long way to helping you choose the most suitable supplements for your health.

Bibliography

Alsanad SM, Williamson EM, Howard RL. (2014). Cancer patients at risk of herb/food supplement-drug interactions: A systematic review. *Phytotherapy Research, 28*(12), 1749–1755. doi:10.1002/ptr.5213.

Binns CW, Lee MK, Lee AH. (2017). Problems and prospects: Public health regulation of dietary supplements. *Annual Review of Public Health, 39*, 403–420. doi:10.1146/annurev-publhealth-040617-013638.

Cadeau C, Fournier A, Mesrine S, Clavel-Chapelon F, Fagherazzi G, Boutron-Ruault M-C. (2016). Vitamin C supplement intake and post-menopausal breast cancer risk: Interaction with dietary vitamin C. *The American Journal of Clinical Nutrition, 104*(1), 228–234. doi:10.3945/ajcn.115.126326.

Caetano BF, de Moura NA, Almeida AP, Dias MC, Sivieri K, Barbisan LF. (2016). Yacon (*Smallanthus sonchifolius*) as a food supplement: Health-promoting benefits of fructooligosaccharides. *Nutrients, 8*(7), 436. doi:10.3390/nu8070436.

de Munter L, Maasland DHE, van den Brandt PA, Kremer B, Schouten LJ. (2015). Vitamin and carotenoid intake and risk of head-neck cancer subtypes in the Netherlands Cohort Study. *The American Journal of Clinical Nutrition, 102*(2), 420–432. doi:10.3945/ajcn.114.106096.

Kim SJ, Zuchniak A, Sohn KJ, *et al.* (2016). Plasma folate, vitamin B-6, and vitamin B-12 and breast cancer risk in BRCA1- and BRCA2-mutation carriers: A prospective study. *The American Journal of Clinical Nutrition, 104*(3), 671–677. doi:10.3945/ajcn.116.133470.

Lefanc F, Tabanca N, Kiss R. (2017). Assessing the anticancer effects associated with food products and/or nutraceuticals using in vitro and in vivo preclinical development-related pharmacological tests. *Seminars in Cancer Biology, 46*, 14–32. doi:10.1016/j.semcancer.2017.06.004.

Mocellin S, Briarava M, Pilati P. (2017). Vitamin B6 and cancer risk: A field synopsis and meta-analysis. *Journal of the National Cancer Institute, 109*(3), djw230. doi:10.1093/jnci/djw230.

Mowry JB, Spyker DA, Cantilena LR Jr, McMillan N, Ford M. (2014). 2013 Annual Report of the American Association of Poison Control Centers' National Poison Data System (NPDS): 31st Annual Report. *Clinical Toxicology, 52*, 1032–1283. Retrieved on December 9, 2019.

New York Attorney General Office. (2019). A.G. Schneiderman asks major retailers to halt sales of certain herbal supplements as DNA tests fail to detect plant materials listed on majority of products tested. Retrieved on December 9, 2019.

Newmaster SG, Grguric M, Shanmughanandhan D, Ramalingam S, Ragupathy S. (2013). DNA barcoding detects contamination and substitution in North American herbal products. *BMC Medicine, 11*, 222.

Office of Dietary Supplements, National Institutes of Health. Making decisions. Retrieved on December 9, 2019.

Playdon MC, Ziegler RG, Sampson JN, *et al.* (2017). Nutritional metabolomics and breast cancer risk in a prospective study. *The American Journal of Clinical Nutrition, 106*(2), 637–649. doi:10.3945/ajcn.116.150912.

Singh P, Yadav RJ, Pandey A. (2005). Utilization of indigenous systems of medicine & homoeopathy in India. *Indian Journal of Medical Research, 122*(2), 137–142.

US Food and Drug Administration. (2005, April). Dietary supplement labeling guide: Chapter VI. Claims. Guidance for Industry. Retrieved on December 9, 2019 from www.fda.gov/food/guidanceregulation/guidancedocumentsregulatoryinformation/dietarysupplements/ucm070613.htm.

US Food and Drug Administration. (2011). FDA 101: Dietary supplements. Retrieved on December 9, 2019 from www.fda.gov/ForConsumers/ConsumerUpdates/ucm050803.htm.

US Food and Drug Administration. (2012). Number of mandatory adverse events reports from the dietary supplement industry entered into CAERS each month. Fiscal Year 2012. Retrieved on December 9, 2019 from www.accessdata.fda.gov/FDATrack/track?program=cfsan&id=CFSAN-OFDCER-Number-of-mandatory-adverse-event-reports-from-dietary-supplement-industry-entered-into-CAERS&fy=2012.

US Food and Drug Administration. (2013, July 16). DMAA in dietary supplements. Retrieved on December 9, 2019 from www.fda.gov/food/dietarysupplements/qadietarysupplements/ucm346576.htm.

US Food and Drug Administration. (2015). Beware of fraudulent dietary supplements. Retrieved on December 9, 2019 from www.fda.gov/for-consumers/consumerupdates/ucm246744.htm.

US Food and Drug Administration, Center for Food Safety and Applied Nutrition. (2007, June 2). Dietary Supplement Current Good Manufacturing Practices (CGMPs) and Interim Final Rule (IFR) Facts. Retrieved on December 9, 2019.

US Food and Drug Administration, Center for Food Safety and Applied Nutrition. (2019). Dietary Supplement Health and Education Act of 1994.

US Pharmacopeial Convention. USP verified dietary supplements. Retrieved on December 9, 2019 from http://www.usp.org/usp-verification-services/usp-verified-dietary-supplements.

Webb PM, Ibiebele TI, Hughes MC, *et al.* (2011). Folate and related micro-nutrients, folate-metabolising genes and risk of ovarian cancer. *European Journal of Clinical Nutrition, 65*(10), 1133–1140. doi:10.1038/ejcn.2011.99.

Whitmore, A. USFDA. Personal communication. Retrieved on December 9, 2019.

Yang W, Ma Y, Smith-Warner S, *et al.* (2019). Calcium intake and survival after colorectal cancer diagnosis. *Clinical Cancer Research, 25*(6), 1980–1988. doi:10.1158/1078-0432.CCR-18-2965.

Chapter 27

Ink with Care

Tattoo is an old practice, which has been in existence since 1800 for religious and cultural purposes. This practice has evolved into fashion and is patronized by people irrespective of the age, race, or social status. As this practice becomes frequent, more questions arise as the inks being used might contain harmful chemicals. The question as to whether tattoo causes cancer is a question researchers have taken a key interest in. Untill now, there is no causal link between tattoo and cancer; however, epidemiological as well as few laboratory studies have indicated that there could be a potential association between tattoo and cancer (Fig. 1).

Black ink is frequently used by tattoo artists and contains high levels of benzo(a)pyrene, a chemical that is listed as a carcinogen by the International Agency for Research on Cancer (IARC). Researchers have expressed concerns since this chemical is capable of initiating cancer development in users. A review study done in 2018 reported 30 cases with observed skin cancer in the tattoos of people. It is yet to be proven if the ink resulted in the formation of the cancer or it was just a coincidence. There is also another case where skin cancer was diagnosed at the chest area of a man covered with tattoos. Although these findings are still correlative, it provides promising rationale for this to be investigated further.

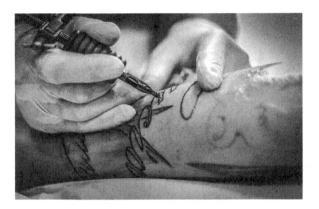

Fig. 1. Tattooing with a black ink

Another chemical found in the ink of tattoos is called titanium dioxide. This chemical has been classified by the IARC as a potential carcinogen and hence has the ability to cause cancer. Titanium dioxide from tattoo inks has been shown to accumulate in the lymph nodes and could create an enabling environment for cancer growth. In a case reported in Australia, doctors were tricked to think a patient had lymphoma but only to realize it was an accumulation of titanium dioxide in her enlarged lymph nodes when detected under the microscope.

There are other chemicals that could be carried into the lymph nodes. The accumulation could cause a reaction with immune cells, resulting in inflammation. It is yet to be scientifically proven if this could result in cancer; however, carcinogens are potential cancer-causing agents and should be used carefully. There is the need to study the long-term effect of these chemicals to provide findings to substantiate the association of tattoo ink with cancer.

There have been cases where skin allergies as a result of these inks have been reported. Most of these allergies cause inflammation, which are breeding grounds for cancer development, although not proven yet. Hepatitis infection is also a growing concern where tattoo artists do not sterilize their instruments before usage. This viral infection is easily transferred via shared needles and body fluids.

There are lots of findings that associate hepatitis with liver cancer hence care should be taken.

The fact that no concrete causal link has been established does not suggest that exposure to tattoo inks could not increase cancer risk. There are correlative associations with chemicals contained in the inks; however, further mechanistic studies are needed to establish a cause and effect relationship. With the confirmation of carcinogenic chemicals in tattoo inks, care should be taken when requesting a tattoo. It will be beneficial to find out if you do not have any preexisting risk factors that will trigger the harmful effects of these chemicals. Regardless, further studies are needed to investigate the mechanistic action of these chemicals on human cells as well as novel means of suppressing their activities. It is highly recommended for chemical regulating authorities to regulate the amount of these chemicals permissible in the inks used for tattoos. Regular checks on tattoo inks will be necessary to ban the products containing harmful chemicals as well as those in high quantities. Although the focus is on clients receiving the body arts, it is possible that the body artists could be exposed to these harmful chemicals. Protective gears are therefore encouraged to be worn to prevent body contact with such chemicals as well as accidental needle pricks and cuts.

Bibliography

Caccavale S, Moscarella E, De Fata Salvatores G, Piccolo V, Russo T, Argenziano G. (2016). When a melanoma is uncovered by a tattoo. *International Journal of Dermatology, 55*(1), 79–80. doi:10.1111/ijd.13124.

Gallè F, Quaranta A, Napoli C, *et al.* (2012). Body art practices and health risks: Young adults' knowledge in two regions of southern Italy. *Annali di igiene: medicina preventiva e di comunità, 24*(6), 535–542.

Juhas E, English JC. (2013). Tattoo-associated complications. *Journal of Pediatric and Adolescent Gynecology, 26*(2), 125–129. doi:10.1016/j.jpag.2012.08.005.

Kazandjieva J, Tsankov N. (2007). Tattoos: Dermatological complications. *Clinics in Dermatology, 25*(4), 375–82.

Kluger N. (2009). Evidence inconclusive regarding tattoos and skin cancer. *Clinical Journal of Oncology Nursing, 13*(3), 260–261. doi:10.1188/09. CJON.259-262.

Kluger N. (2015). Contraindications for tattooing. *Current Problems in Dermatology, 48*, 76–87. doi:10.1159/000369189.

Kluger N. (2019). An update on cutaneous complications of permanent tattooing. *Expert Review of Clinical Immunology, 15*(11), 1135–1143. doi: 10.1080/1744666X.2020.1676732.

Kluger N, Douvin D, Dupuis-Fourdan F, Doumecq-Lacoste JM, Descamps V. (2017). Keratoacanthomas on recent tattoos: Two cases. *Annales de Dermatologie et de Vénéréologie, 144*(12), 776–783. doi:10.1016/j.annder. 2017.10.006.

Kluger N, Koskenmies S, Jeskanen L, Övermark M, Saksela O. (2014). Melanoma on tattoos: Two Finnish cases. *Acta Dermato-Venereologica, 94*(3), 325–326. doi:10.2340/00015555-1705.

Laux P, Tralau T, Tentschert J, *et al.* (2016). A medical-toxicological view of tattooing. *Lancet, 387*(10016), 395–402. doi:10.1016/S0140-6736(15) 60215-X.

Lerche CM, Heerfordt IM, Serup J, Poulsen T, Wulf HC. (2017). Red tattoos, ultraviolet radiation and skin cancer in mice. *Experimental Dermatology, 26*, 1091–1096. doi:10.1111/exd.13383.

Manganoni AM, Sereni E, Pata G, *et al.* (2014). Pigmentation of axillary sentinel nodes from extensive skin tattoo mimics metastatic melanoma: Case report. *International Journal of Dermatology, 53*(6), 773–776. doi:10.1111/ijd.12417.

Marchesi A, Parodi PC, Brioschi M, *et al.* (2014). Tattoo ink-related cutaneous pseudolymphoma: A rare but significant complication. Case report and review of the literature. *Aesthetic Plastic Surgery, 38*(2), 471–478. doi:10.1007/s00266-014-0287-5.

Naeini FF, Pourazizi M, Abtahi-Naeini B, Saffaei A, Bagheri F. (2017). Looking beyond the cosmetic tattoo lesion near the eyebrow: Screening the lungs. *Journal of Postgraduate Medicine, 63*(2), 132–134. doi:10.4103/ 0022-3859.201421.

Navrazhina K, Goldman B, Leger MC. (2018). Atypical intraepidermal melanocytic proliferation masked by a tattoo: Implications for tattoo artists and public health campaigns. *Cureus, 10*(7), e2975. doi:10.7759/cureus.2975.

Paprottka FJ, Krezdorn N, Narwan M, *et al.* (2017). Trendy tattoos-maybe a serious health risk? *Aesthetic Plastic Surgery, 42*, 310–321. doi:10.1007/ s00266-017-1002-0.

Quaranta A, Napoli C, Fasano F, Montagna C, Caggiano G, Montagna MT. (2011). Body piercing and tattoos: A survey on young adults' knowledge of the risks and practices in body art. *BMC Public Health, 11*, 774. doi:10.1186/1471-2458-11-774.

Serup J, Carlsen KH, Sepehri M. (2015). Tattoo complaints and complications: Diagnosis and clinical spectrum. *Current Problems in Dermatology, 48*, 48–60. doi:10.1159/000369645.

Soran A, Menekse E, Kanbour-Shakir A, *et al.* (2017). The importance of tattoo pigment in sentinel lymph nodes. *Breast Disease, 37*(2), 73–76. doi:10.3233/BD-170282.

Zafar A, Mustafa M, Chapman M. (2012). Colorectal polyps: When should we tattoo? *Surgical Endoscopy, 26*(11), 3264–3266. doi:10.1007/s00464-012-2335-z.

Chapter 28

Modern Trends in Cancer Therapeutics

Over the years, cancer treatments have evolved so much. This is as a result of intensive research directed to discovering new targets for treatments as well as early diagnosis. The conventional treatments for various types of cancer have been chemotherapy, radiotherapy, and surgery. Although most patients respond very well initially, a huge number of these patients return to the clinic with tumor recurrence and ultimately become resistant to further treatment. This has been the motivation toward the discovery of new targets to impact the overall survival of patients.

Patients' response to cancer treatments is dependent on a couple of factors. Oncologists take into consideration such factors in the planning of treatment regimen for these patients. For example, the age, type of cancer, tumor stage, and grade are all key players in planning an effective treatment. There are instances where a patient will need more than one combination of treatments such as mostly seen with ovarian cancer patients — surgical debulking with chemotherapeutic agents (standard treatment). There are times the tumor is too large to be taken out by surgery hence chemotherapy (neoadjuvant) is given to shrink the size before surgery is done to remove it. There

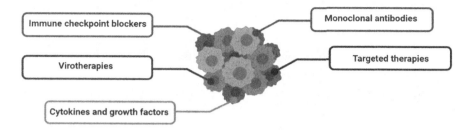

Fig. 1. Types of alternative treatments that harness the immune system to fight cancer

are other chemotherapeutic agents (adjuvant) that are given after surgery to prevent possible recurrence.

The ultimate goal of chemotherapy is to destroy cells that grow uncontrollably. However, these agents also target normal cells and end up causing massive toxicities to the patients. In some cases, these patients die from the adverse side effects but not the cancer itself. This has led to other alternative treatments such as hormonal therapy (mostly used in prostate, uterine, and breast cancers), targeted small therapies (using small molecules to target genes), immunotherapy (where the immune cells are boosted to kill the cancer cells and has shown promise in melanoma), and supportive drugs [Allopurinol (Zyloprim), Rasburicase (Fasturtec), Amifostine (Ethyol), Folinic acid (leucovorin), Dexrazoxane (Zinecard)] to minimize side effects from other cancer treatments (Fig. 1).

In the last decade, immunotherapy has revolutionized cancer treatments, leading to a huge investment in this area of research. During cancer development, the immune system is suppressed to enable the cancer to thrive and spread to other parts of the body. Harnessing the immune system therefore presents as a promising approach to fighting these cancer cells while minimizing toxicities. Immunotherapy is used to achieve several purposes such as delivering radioisotopes or toxins to the cancer cells, slowing down or stopping cancer growth, and halting the spread of the cancer to other parts of the body.

There are different types of immunotherapies and which one to be used depends on the type of cancer.

1. Immune checkpoint blockers: The cancer cells are so smart that they can put brakes on the immune cells (T cells). This makes the T cells see the cancer cells as part of the human body so do not attack them. These brakes are called the checkpoint proteins. There are several of these proteins; however, the most characterized ones are PD-1 (expressed on activated T cells), PDL1 (mostly expressed on the tumor), and CTLA-4 (expressed on activated T cells). Checkpoint blockers are monoclonal antibodies that bind to these brakes and block their inhibitory influence, thus, releasing the T cells to fight and kill the cancer cells. There are FDA-approved checkpoint blockers that have proven to be clinically relevant in melanoma, non-small cell lung cancer, Hodgkin's lymphoma, and kidney cancers. Examples of these are atezolizumab (Tecentriq), pembrolizumab (Keytruda), and nivolumab (Opdivo) that target PD-1 or PD-L1 and ipilimumab (Yervoy) that targets CTLA-4. There are instances where a combination of these treatments have a significant tumor killing efficiency compared with individual treatments.

2. Monoclonal antibodies: These are developed against proteins that are responsible for cancer growth. These antibodies function by binding and attaching to the target proteins. Once attached, they block growth signals responsible for tumor growth as well as receptors that transit these signals. Also, they are used to deliver secret weapons (toxins, viruses, radioisotopes) to specific cancer tissues. Examples of monoclonal antibodies include Rituximab (Rituxan) that is used for the treatment of non-Hodgkin lymphoma and chronic lymphocytic leukemia (CLL), Bevacizumab (Avastin) that is used to target vascular endothelial growth factor (VEGF) receptor proteins in ovarian, colorectal, and cervical cancers, Cetuximab (Erbitux) for targeting epidermal growth factor receptor (EGFR) proteins in colorectal and head-and-neck cancers, and Trastuzumab (Herceptin) for targeting HER2 positive breast cancers.

3. Conjugated monoclonal antibodies: These are antibodies that are used to deliver radioactive isotopes or chemotherapeutic agents. This approach is intended to increase the specificity of treatment and minimize toxicities. In the treatment of non-Hodgkin lymphoma, a monoclonal antibody, Ibritumomab (Zevalin) is tagged with radioactive isotope yttrium-90. Monoclonal antibodies could also be tagged with drugs, which is the case of Brentuximab vedotin (Adcetris) used in the treatment of Hodgkin lymphoma. Trastuzumab emtansine (Kadcyla or T-DM1) is another example of antibody–drug conjugate that has been used in the treatment of HER2 positive metastatic breast cancer.

4. Cytokines and growth factors immunotherapies: There are instances where nonspecific immunotherapies could be used for the treatment of cancer. Cytokines and growth factors are examples of these approaches. Cytokines are chemicals secreted by cells to help in the fighting of diseases such as cancer. Interferon alfa (Intron A, Wellferon) has shown great promise in the treatment of blood cancers. Interleukin-2 (Proleukin) has also shown promise in the treatment of kidney cancer and melanoma. Blood growth factors such as granulocyte colony-stimulating factor (G-CSF) and granulocyte-macrophage colony-stimulating factor (GM-CSF) help boost the immune system for cancer treatment.

5. Virotherapy: Recently, researchers are utilizing viruses to fight cancers. These viruses are known as oncolytic viruses. Oncolytic viruses are used to produce an immunostimulating environment to help in the killing of cancer cells. These viruses have shown promise in non-small cell lung cancer, glioblastoma, ovarian cancers, among others. Dr. John Bell at the Ottawa Hospital Research Institute (OHRI), Ottawa, Canada, oversees a team that specializes in manufacturing oncolytic viruses for cancer treatment. There are other laboratories across the world that are also doing amazing work in this field.

Targeted therapies utilize small molecules to target genes responsible for cancer growth. These molecules inhibit the signals that fuel the growth of the cancer cells. Examples of these therapies include the following:

1. Apoptosis-inducing drugs: These drugs interact with enzymes and proteins which reactivate the signals involved with inducing programmed cell death (apoptosis). Examples are Olaparib (Lynparza) that inhibits poly ADP-ribose polymerase (PARP), Bortezomib (Velcade) that inhibits proteasomes, and Oblimersen (Genasense) that inhibits BCL2 (a cancer survival protein).
2. Tyrosine kinase inhibitors: Tyrosine kinases are enzymes responsible for sending growth signals for cancer development. Inhibiting these signals therefore halts growth signal transmission resulting in cancer cell death. Examples are Imatinib (Gleevec) and Gefitinib (Iressa).
3. Angiogenesis inhibitors: Developing new blood vessels is key for tumor growth and survival. This happens when VEGF binds to its receptor on the cancer cells. Thus, inhibiting this process could offer a therapeutic approach to kill the cancer cells. There are clinically proven inhibitors that target either the growth factor or its receptor: Bevacizumab (Avastin), Sunitinib (Sutent), and Thalidomide (Thalomid).
4. mTOR inhibitors: mTOR plays a huge role in controlling cell division and growth. When mTOR is defective, it leads to uncontrolled growth of cells that contribute to cancer development. Inhibiting such process could offer therapeutic advantages to cancer patients. Examples of these inhibitors are emsirolimus (Torisel) and everolimus (Afinitor).

Cancer vaccines are made up of the patients' cancer cells, antigens, or DNA with the intention of stimulating the immune system to fight cancer. The immune response generated after the vaccine injection specifically recognizes the antigens from the tumor. Examples of these include whole tumor vaccines (the whole tumor is used), antigen vaccines (only antigens from the cancer are used), and DNA vaccines (the DNA is isolated from the cancer of the patient). There are instances where the patients' dendritic cells (cells that present antigens to the tumor killing cells) are isolated and educated to recognize specific antigens on the patients' tumor. Once this is done, the reeducated dendritic cells are reintroduced into the patient's body to fight the tumor. This is called the dendritic cell vaccine.

Although immunotherapy has shown tremendous improvement in some types of cancers, there are side effects associated ranging from mild to severe. Always discuss with your oncologist to know which of these treatments will work best for you since individual response is different. There are clinical trials that recruit patients to test some of these new discoveries and one could discuss with his or her clinician to decide whether to enroll or not. In the coming years, it is expected that most of the cancer treatments will be patient-tailored, also known as precision medicine. Thus, the patient's tumor will be sequenced and mutated genes detected. Treatments will therefore be generated to specifically target these genes, taking into consideration the patient's medical history. However, the technologies involved will mean such treatments will be expensive and less accessible. In our quest to finding the magic bullet to cancer, we should also consider how such treatments will be made accessible to all patients irrespective of their economic status.

Bibliography

Akinleye A, Rasool Z. (2019). Immune checkpoint inhibitors of PD-L1 as cancer therapeutics. *Journal of Hematology & Oncology, 12,* 92. doi:10.1186/s13045-019-0779-5.

Alessandrini F, Menotti L, Avitabile E, *et al.* (2019). Eradication of glioblastoma by immuno-virotherapy with a retargeted oncolytic HSV in a preclinical model. *Oncogene, 38,* 4467–4479. doi:10.1038/s41388-019-0737-2.

American Cancer Society. (2008, March 18). *Immunotherapy.* Atlanta, GA: American Cancer Society.

Breastcancer.org. (2016, May 16). HER2 Status. Retrieved from http://www.breastcancer.org/symptoms/diagnosis/her2.

Chang E, Sabichi AL, Kramer JR, *et al.* (2018). Nivolumab treatment for cancers in the HIV-infected population. *Journal of Immunotherapy (Hagerstown, MD. : 1997)*, *41*(8), 379–383. doi:10.1097/CJI.0000000000000240.

De Giorgi U, Cartenì G, Giannarelli D, *et al.* (2018). Safety and efficacy of nivolumab for metastatic renal cell carcinoma: Real-world results from an expanded access program. *BJU International*, *123*, 98–105. doi:10.1111/bju.14461.

Hodi FS, Chesney J, Pavlick AC, *et al.* (2016). Combined nivolumab and ipilimumab versus ipilimumab alone in patients with advanced melanoma: 2-year overall survival outcomes in a multicentre, randomised, controlled, phase 2 trial. *The Lancet Oncology*, *17*(11), 1558–1568. doi:10.1016/S1470-2045(16)30366-7.

https://www.cancer.ca/en/cancer-information. Retrieved on October 30, 2019.

Joseph RW, Chatta G, Vaishampayan U. (2017). Nivolumab treatment for advanced renal cell carcinoma: Considerations for clinical practice. *Urologic Oncology*, *35*(4), 142–148. doi:10.1016/j.urolonc.2017.01.017.

Kamata T, Suzuki A, Mise N, *et al.* (2016). Blockade of programmed death-1/programmed death ligand pathway enhances the antitumor immunity of human invariant natural killer T cells. *Cancer Immunology, Immunotherapy: CII*, *65*(12), 1477–1489. doi:10.1007/s00262-016-1901-y.

Kellish P, Shabashvili D, Rahman MM, *et al.* (2019). Oncolytic virotherapy for small-cell lung cancer induces immune infiltration and prolongs survival. *The Journal of Clinical Investigation*, *129*(6), 2279–2292. doi:10.1172/JCI121323.

Khan KD, Emmanouilides C, Benson DM Jr, *et al.* (2006). A phase 2 study of rituximab in combination with recombinant interleukin-2 for rituximab-refractory indolent non-Hodgkin's lymphoma. *Clinical Cancer Research: An Official Journal of the American Association for Cancer Research*, *12*(23), 7046–7053. doi:10.1158/1078-0432.CCR-06-1571.

Kimura H, Sone T, Murata A, *et al.* (2017). Long-lasting shrinkage in tumor mass after discontinuation of nivolumab treatment. *Lung Cancer, 108*, 7–8. doi:10.1016/j.lungcan.2017.02.013.

Kudo T, Hamamoto Y, Kato K, *et al.* (2017). Nivolumab treatment for oesophageal squamous-cell carcinoma: An open-label, multicentre, phase 2 trial. *Lancet*, *18*(5), 631–639. doi:10.1016/S1470-2045(17)30181-X.

Lee SM, Chow LQ. (2014). A new addition to the PD-1 checkpoint inhibitors for non-small cell lung cancer-the anti-PDL1 antibody-MEDI4736.

Translational Lung Cancer Research, *3*(6), 408–410. doi:10.3978/j. issn.2218-6751.2014.11.10.

Lynch TJ, Bondarenko I, Luft A, *et al.* (2012). Ipilimumab in combination with paclitaxel and carboplatin as first-line treatment in stage IIIB/IV non-small-cell lung cancer: Results from a randomized, double-blind, multicenter phase II study. *Journal of Clinical Oncology: Official Journal of the American Society of Clinical Oncology*, *30*(17), 2046–2054. doi:10.1200/ JCO.2011.38.4032.

McDermott D, Haanen J, Chen T-T, Lorigan P, O'Day S, MDX010-20 Investigators. (2013). Efficacy and safety of ipilimumab in metastatic melanoma patients surviving more than 2 years following treatment in a phase III trial (MDX010-20). *Annals of Oncology*, *24*(10), 2694–2698. doi:10.1093/annonc/mdt291.

Monk BJ, Minion LE, Coleman RL. (2016). Anti-angiogenic agents in ovarian cancer: Past, present, and future. *Annals of Oncology: Official Journal of the European Society for Medical Oncology*, *27* (Suppl. 1), i33–i39. doi:10.1093/annonc/mdw093.

National Cancer Institute. (2014, April 25). *Targeted cancer therapies*. Bethesda: National Cancer Institute. Retrieved from http://www.cancer.gov/about-cancer/treatment/types/targeted-therapies/targeted-therapies-fact-sheet.

Nonomura C, Otsuka M, Kondou R, *et al.* (2019), Identification of a neo-antigen epitope in a melanoma patient with good response to anti-PD-1 antibody therapy, *Immunology Letters.* doi:10.1016/j.imlet.2019.02.004.

Pan Y-A, Su N-W, Leu Y-S. (2019). Anti-PDL1 immunotherapy as a radiosensitizer on treating advanced recurrent oropharyngeal squamous cell carcinoma. *Ear, Nose & Throat Journal.* doi:10.1177/0145561319881565.

Pi G, He H, Bi J, *et al.* (2016). Efficacy of short-term nivolumab treatment in a Chinese patient with relapsed advanced-stage lung squamous cell carcinoma: A case report. *Medicine*, *95*(40), e5077. doi:10.1097/ MD.0000000000005077.

Postow MA, Manuel M, Wong P, *et al.* (2015). Peripheral T cell receptor diversity is associated with clinical outcomes following ipilimumab treatment in metastatic melanoma. *Journal for Immunotherapy of Cancer*, *3*, 23. doi:10.1186/s40425-015-0070-4.

Qi N, Li F, Li X, Kang H, Zhao H, Du N. (2016). Combination use of paclitaxel and avastin enhances treatment effect for the NSCLC patients with malignant pleural effusion. *Medicine*, *95*(47), e5392. doi:10.1097/ MD.0000000000005392.

Rini BI, Halabi S, Taylor J, Small EJ, Schilsky RL, Cancer and Leukemia Group B. (2004). Cancer and Leukemia Group B 90206: A randomized phase III trial of interferon-alpha or interferon-alpha plus anti-vascular endothelial growth factor antibody (bevacizumab) in metastatic renal cell carcinoma. *Clinical Cancer Research: An Official Journal of the American Association for Cancer Research*, 10(8), 2584–2586.

Simeone E, Grimaldi AM, Ascierto PA. (2015). Anti-PD1 and anti-PD-L1 in the treatment of metastatic melanoma. *Melanoma Management*, 2(1), 41–50. doi:10.2217/mmt.14.30.

Suksanpaisan L, Xu R, Tesfay MZ, *et al.* (2018). Preclinical development of oncolytic immunovirotherapy for treatment of HPVPOS cancers. *Molecular Therapy Oncolytics, 10*, 1–13. doi:10.1016/j.omto.2018.05.001.

Twumasi-Boateng K, Pettigrew JL, Kwok YYE. *et al.* (2018). Oncolytic viruses as engineering platforms for combination immunotherapy. *Nature Reviews Cancer, 18*, 419–432. doi:10.1038/s41568-018-0009-4.

Chapter 29

Conclusion

There are people out there who make money out of false advertisements regarding causes and treatments for cancer. Some of these claims put fear into people and unfortunately lure them into believing these false claims. Until you believe anything, it's imperative to have a discussion with experts to sieve the myths from the facts. Having open discussions with your healthcare professionals will provide you the ability to think through advertisements before making a decision, especially in the case of dietary supplements. Also, desist from forwarding hoax messages and emails since these acts make you a culprit in propagating falsehood. Many have lost their lives due to wrong decisions made based on such falsehood.

In addition to researchers, there are other stakeholders who are key in the fight against cancer. Many thanks to all funding agencies who consistently support medical research especially cancer research. The findings from these research activities are the sources of hope for many patients including those living with cancer. The patients who willingly consent to donating their body tissues and fluids for research are the real MVPs. Their selfless efforts have resulted in the development of novel therapies for the service of mankind. The sad thing is, most of these wonderful patients do not even live to see or benefit from such breakthrough treatments.

The complexities of cancer cannot be underestimated; however, knowing the facts from the myths could help appreciate the gift of life and the need to stay healthy. Although we might not have total control on inherited mutated genes, pragmatic steps could be taken to lower the risk of developing cancer. The complex nature of cancer demands a multidisciplinary approach to fighting it. Thus, there is the need for artificial intelligence/machine learning and other advanced technologies in cancer research. This should not only be the responsibility of biology-inclined scientists; other professionals such as engineers, IT experts, mathematicians, and physicists could bring their expertise on board for a collective fight. The battle will indeed be difficult; however, with determination, honesty, and transparency, the fight against cancer will be a successful one.

About the Author

Dr. Meshach Asare-Werehene is a clinical diagnostic and immuno-oncology expert based in Ottawa, Canada. As the team lead of the cancer immunology program in the Tsang lab, Department of Gynecology and Obstetrics, The Ottawa Hospital, he focuses on the discovery of novel diagnostic and therapeutic modalities for chemoresistant ovarian cancer patients. Through his cutting-edge research and clinical collaboration locally and internationally, he has published and presented novel findings on ovarian cancer in prestigious peer-reviewed journals and at international conferences. His finding that a protein called gelsolin in the blood could be used as an early diagnostic tool for ovarian cancer patients has attracted international audience and is being further developed for clinical use. Dr. Asare-Werehene holds a Ph.D. in Medicine from the University of Ottawa, Canada and has also received clinical and research trainings from the University of Nottingham, UK and Kwame Nkrumah University of Science and Technology (KNUST), Ghana. He has received advanced trainings in the field of oncology including breast cancer diagnosis and management from Yale School of Medicine, USA via Coursera.

Dr. Asare-Werehene is a member of the Society for the Study of Reproduction (SSR) and the International Society for Precision Cancer Medicine (ISPCM). He is a Christian, an avid reader and writer, a social commentator and married to Dr. Afrakoma Afriyie-Asante, an immunologist and clinical diagnostic expert.

Index